Praise for *Train Your Brain to Beat Chronic Pain*

"I have read many books about chronic pain, and this one is the most useful! Dr. Hunt's insights are grounded in scientific expertise as well as her own experience, which really resonated with me. I am familiar with (and already use) some of the ideas in this book, but see new strategies I am eager to try for solving the chronic pain puzzle."
—Lou N., Baltimore

"A comprehensive and powerful guide to overcoming chronic pain. Dr. Hunt discusses mental training techniques and integrative care plans for conquering pain that can be easy to implement. This book is an amazing resource for patients with chronic health conditions who are looking to get started on managing their pain in tangible ways."
—Dana DiRenzo, MD, MHS, Assistant Professor of Clinical Medicine (Rheumatology), Penn Medicine

"Accessible, warm, and compassionate, this book combines personal and clinical experience with up-to-date scientific research to offer a comprehensive toolkit for moving beyond chronic pain. The book is filled with information and clearly presented exercises that can help anyone suffering from chronic pain to lead a fuller, more meaningful, less painful life."
—Ronald D. Siegel, PsyD, author of *The Extraordinary Gift of Being Ordinary*

"Dr. Hunt provides an essential roadmap for navigating the twists and turns of daily life with chronic pain and finding a new path forward. Grounded in a modern neuroscience of pain, this book accentuates the importance of the mind–body connection. From meditation exercises to sleep health habits to insurance reimbursement tips, this book abounds with practical recommendations that will empower you to effectively manage your pain and flourish in the process."
—Patrick H. Finan, PhD, Harold Carron Professor of Anesthesiology, University of Virginia School of Medicine

TRAIN YOUR BRAIN
TO BEAT CHRONIC PAIN

TRAIN YOUR BRAIN TO BEAT CHRONIC PAIN

How to Harness the Power
of the Mind–Body Connection

Carly Hunt, PhD

𝕊𝕡

THE GUILFORD PRESS
New York   London

Printed in the United States of America

For product and safety concerns within the EU, please contact GPSR@taylorandfrancis.com,
Taylor & Francis Verlag GmbH, Kaufingerstraße 24, 80331 München, Germany.

Last digit is print number: 9 8 7 6 5 4 3 2 1

This publication is intended to provide helpful and informative material. It is not intended to
diagnose, treat, cure, or prevent any health problem or condition, nor is it intended to replace
the advice of a health professional. No action should be taken based solely on the contents of
this book. Always consult your physician or qualified health care professional on any matters
regarding your health and before adopting any suggestions in this book or drawing inferences
from it.

The author and publisher specifically disclaim all responsibility for any liability, loss, or
risk, personal or otherwise, which is incurred as a consequence, directly or indirectly, from
the use or application of any contents of this book.

Any and all product names referenced within this book are the trademarks of their
respective owners. Always read all information provided by the manufacturers' product labels
before using their products. The author and publisher are not responsible for claims made by
manufacturers.

Library of Congress Cataloging-in-Publication Data

Names: Hunt, Carly author
Title: Train your brain to beat chronic pain : how to harness the power of
   the mind-body connection / Carly Hunt.
Description: New York : The Guilford Press, [2026] | Includes
   bibliographical references and index.
Identifiers: LCCN 2025030295 | ISBN 9781462552962 paperback |
   ISBN 9781462558520 hardcover
Subjects: LCSH: Chronic pain—Treatment | Chronic pain—Psychological
   aspects | Mind and body | Mental healing
Classification: LCC RB127.5.C48 H86 2026
LC record available at https://lccn.loc.gov/2025030295

To my wonderful family,
and to all people who live with chronic pain

Contents

Acknowledgments

So many have been benefactors to me in my work and life. This book is one of the many ways I stand on their shoulders.

First, to my extraordinarily loving and supportive parents—thank you for your love, encouragement, and guidance through the joyful and difficult times in my life. You've made this book possible, and I love you.

To my husband, Brian—I'm so lucky to have met such a wonderful partner and friend. I'm so grateful for your love, encouragement, sense of humor, and presence in my life. From your intellectual input, to unloading the dishwasher for quite literally the millionth time, to helping me believe in myself, you've helped make this book come to life. I love you.

To my son, Aidan—you made me a mother. You're always on an adventure, and I thank you for showing me what it means to be present, joyful, and in awe of this life every day. I'm so proud of you and love you. To my daughter Maggie—you're so new, yet so wise. Thank you for joining us in this world. I love you so.

To my wonderful family: Kasie, Matt, Mars, and Grey; Alonzo and Jacqueline Keathley; Lenore Hunt; Lisa, Ray, and Jenna; John and George; Craig, Laura, Davis, Jan, and Tom; Kathy and Rick, Arnie, and my wonderful cousins and aunts and uncles—thank you for your generosity, love, and support.

To my fantastic editors, Chris Benton and Kitty Moore, who truly made this process fun—I feel so lucky to have been able to work with you. Thank you for everything.

To my wonderful Johns Hopkins colleagues and collaborators: Drs. Patrick Finan, Michael Smith, Jennifer Haythornthwaite, Chung Jung Mun, Janelle Letzen, Matthew Reid, Catlin DuPont, Jennifer Ellis, Janelle Coughlin, Neda Gould, Dana Direnzo, and Ceyda Sayalı—thank you so much for your exceptional collegiality, friendship, and support in making this book happen.

Dr. Elizabeth Sauber—thank you so much for helping to improve parts of this book and for your friendship.

Dr. Mary Ann Hoffman—thank you so much for your unwavering support as I battled a chronic pain condition while trying to finish graduate school, not to mention your kindness and generosity in general.

To Dr. David Seminowicz, Dr. Joe Tatta, DPT, Dr. Yoni Ashar, and Carmen Roberts, MS, RD, LDN—thank you for your generous contributions in reviewing sections of this text.

To the many mentors who've offered me so much wisdom and guidance on my way through academia and beyond: Dr. Fathali Moghaddam, Dr. Tomas Pruzinsky, Wilson Hurley, and Drs. Clara Hill, Charles Gelso, Dennis Kivlighan, and Barbara Thompson.

Lastly, I would like to thank the meditation teachers and groups that have offered me so much wisdom and guidance: Tara Brach, Jack Kornfield, Shell Fischer, Mary Grace Orr, Ruth King, and the Mind & Life Institute—you've impacted me in countless ways, including my ability to write this book.

Introduction

As I write this I think back to when I started my postdoctoral fellowship training in biobehavioral pain research at the Johns Hopkins School of Medicine. I was sitting in a small auditorium for the weekly pain research seminar; it was packed with some of the most well-regarded pain researchers and clinicians in the world. The presenter that day was a pediatric pain specialist, and I choked back tears as he read a poem written by one of his patients about how her pain came after her in the night, like a tiger—violent, scary, and mean. I hid my sadness in an effort to look like the other scientists around me—collected, focused, competent. Yet I was someone who'd lived with intermittent pain my whole life in the wake of a rare childhood illness, and then with unrelenting, intractable, 8-out-of-10 pain during a period of intense stress in my late 20s. During that latter period, I never felt the urge to escape via suicide, but I had a glimpse into why chronic pain leads some to take their own lives.[1]

Before starting my fellowship, I'd already found a way out of treatment-resistant pain and become pain free—something that, during the peak of my chronic pain disorder, I wasn't sure I'd ever achieve. My journey into healing was multifaceted and unique to me—a key principle of pain treatment that I'll discuss in this book. I tried nearly

---

[1] If you're ever in crisis and need to speak with a counselor immediately, dial 988.

everything—medications, injections of various sorts, supplements, acupuncture, yoga, meditation, spinal manipulation, exercise, dietary changes, psychotherapy, physical therapy, functional medicine, and other major lifestyle modifications. Some medications were very helpful, at times, as part of my journey toward feeling better. Yet the most helpful strategies, in my view, were staying active, seeing a chiropractor, and getting the benefits of functional medicine, nutrition therapy, and long-term psychotherapy. The last plan I undertook was divorcing myself from several unhealthy things in my life, including (1) my husband, (2) people pleasing, and (3) self-criticism. Although avoiding numbers 2 and 3 is still my life's work, I'm free; I notice them when they're happening and then try another way. I'm now remarried to a wonderful partner, live an active life, work full time, and have two young kids. But getting to this point wasn't easy. And I actively engage in a variety of health behaviors to stay pain free.

It's possible that my journey into intermittent and then intractable pain all started with a medical trauma that occurred when I was six years old. One night I awoke to excruciating abdominal pain, which the pediatrician misdiagnosed as the flu. After 48 hours of agony, I went into shock and was rushed to the ER. Exploratory surgery revealed a twisted small intestine and several feet of dead tissue, which was surgically removed along with a nonviable ileocecal valve, an important sphincter muscle that keeps harmful bacteria from overgrowing. Although I was too young to understand, I nearly died. Two years later I experienced a second blockage, emergency surgery, and hospitalization. In the wake of these procedures, I was in intermittent pain throughout childhood and adolescence, even though my internal injuries had healed. Gastroenterologists had varying explanations for why I still had pain. Research shows that early traumatic experiences sensitize the nervous system, putting it on high alert to detect and respond to threats. Likely, this sensitization was at play for me. I'll talk more about nervous system sensitization and trauma and how to address them later in this book.

Fast forward to my early 20s, when I became romantically involved with a fellow graduate student who I knew deep down used alcohol a little bit too much. Yet my ego had organized itself around being the agreeable, accommodating, nice, and unproblematic person who selflessly supported others. So I didn't really allow myself to feel upset about it. It's obvious to me now how this is exactly the type of environment in which addiction plants its seed. As the relationship progressed, I tried harder and harder to suppress my needs and any conscious recognition of the deeply problematic aspects of our relationship. Episodic migraines were a warning signal.

Then a day came when I experienced explosive head and shoulder pain that wouldn't abate. For the ensuing year I was surviving life 15 minutes at a time. My nervous system became so sensitive that I could hardly tolerate wearing a button-down shirt. The medical term for this is *allodynia*, where pain is felt in response to something that normally doesn't provoke pain. Overhead light and normal noise from the television would make me uncomfortable (hypersensitivity to light and sound often accompany allodynia). I was in a dangerous situation (a toxic relationship), and since I wasn't listening to my emotions, my body started to scream. As discussed in Chapter 1, the whole point of pain is to warn us of danger and motivate us to escape. Dangers aren't just physical, they can be emotional, social, and environmental as well. Although I would have preferred a different past, I thank my body for what it did for me; it forced me to pay attention to important threats in my life and to act. Securing healthy interpersonal relationships is an integral part of pain management, which I'll talk more about in this book.

I laugh because when I went back to see one of my pain specialists who'd been giving me nerve blocks and Botox on and off for months, I mentioned that I'd started feeling better and that I had new medical insurance because I'd gotten divorced. She quipped, "It's probably because you got rid of your husband."

Most pain clinicians, who appear so focused on offering you medical interventions, know what the research confirms: pain is a biopsychosocial phenomenon, meaning that biological, social, and psychological factors are all involved in causing and curing pain. They may not be as equipped to help you with all the aspects of pain given their training, but they should support your efforts in addressing them. This book is going to help you do just that.

It's possible to beat chronic pain. Around the world, countless people have done it. I've done it and you can too. Congratulations on your persistence in searching for pain relief. The fact that you've picked up this book shows that you care about your well-being and that part of you trusts that healing is within your reach. Join me as we explore the modern neuroscientific understanding of pain, followed by evidence-based strategies that logically follow from that understanding, which you can start using today. Much of what I write in this book I wish I had known during the peak of my own pain problem. I'm glad you're here!

Your Pain Is Real

I want to emphasize first and foremost that your pain, and all pain, is real. If clinicians, friends, or family members have expressed doubt about how much pain you have or suggest that it's "all in your head," you're not alone. I mention this now because I'm going to discuss the role of the brain in the pain experience. It's vital to understand that the brain is not the mind. During each moment of our lives, the brain is engaged in a truly staggering amount of information processing that happens completely outside of our conscious awareness. A tragedy of the chronic pain experience is the messaging that one's pain is "psychological," that is, without real substance. These messages are invalidating, to say the least, and antithetical to healing. Pain isn't "all in your head," and there's nothing wrong with you for having chronic pain.

This Book Is for You If . . .

- You've been living with persistent pain for at least three months and you're looking for drug-free ways to relieve it;
- You've been diagnosed with a chronic health condition that involves pain, such as fibromyalgia, arthritis, irritable bowel syndrome, or an autoimmune condition;
- You've had an injury and, although doctors and physical therapists have told you your body has healed, you still have pain;
- Your chronic pain arose seemingly out of nowhere, perhaps during a stressful time in your life;
- You've had surgeries or procedures that were supposed to relieve your pain but they failed;

- You had surgery of any sort and ended up with chronic pain afterward;

- You've been told that your pain will never subside or fully go away;

- You want to know the latest information about chronic pain science and how it can help you;

- You're ready to make some major lifestyle changes to promote pain relief;

- You're interested in practicing mental training techniques for pain relief; and

- You want to learn more about integrative pain care (combining multiple treatment approaches in a coordinated way), the recommended approach for chronic pain management.

How to Use This Book

You have chronic pain, and you're not alone. At least 20 percent of the global population suffers from chronic pain. If you're a young person know that other young people experience chronic pain too. It has complex, multifactorial causes and manifestations, and no two people with chronic pain are exactly alike. That's part of what makes pain treatment so challenging. Research is not definitive about who will benefit from which type of treatment, in what combination, and in what order. Pain scientists' understanding of chronic pain is also evolving rapidly. It was only in the past few decades that chronic pain came to be viewed as something that can be a health condition in and of itself, rather than a reflection of some underlying disease or structural problem in the body.

Research suggests that pain can be lowered significantly or eliminated by actively taking charge of your pain problem and engaging in science-backed psychological and behavioral strategies. I'm going to present those to you in this book. Although the Western medical system makes it seem like people experience good health by passively accepting treatments delivered by seemingly all-knowing, all-powerful physicians, when it comes to chronic pain (particularly the variety that has no identifiable underlying disease), nothing could be further from the truth. You are the expert on your own experience and life. In this book I'll be inviting you to reflect on your experience from several angles and to actively apply science-backed mental and behavioral techniques that may help address your unique experience of chronic pain. I'll help you

- Learn about the neuroscience of pain (Chapter 1);
- Take stock of things in your life that may be making your pain worse (Chapter 2);
- Identify sources of joy and meaning that can help lower pain (Chapter 3);
- Understand and implement new behaviors and mental training techniques that lower pain (Chapters 4–13);
- Learn about integrative pain care (Chapter 14); and
- Move forward with a plan (Chapter 15).

Think of a personalized pain relief plan like a recipe, and yours is unique. Treatment approaches, which range from the conventional (medications, injections, surgeries) to brain-retraining techniques covered in this book, fundamentally important health behaviors (optimizing your sleep and nutrition), and complementary medicine (acupuncture, light therapy), constitute pain-relief "ingredients." No matter how much or how little your pain condition requires or benefits from conventional medical approaches (medications, injections, and the like), to feel as well as you possibly can, it is essential to adopt mental and behavioral treatment strategies that we know help lower pain. I'm going to help you understand how brain retraining and lifestyle changes *impact pain neurophysiology:* these aren't simply strategies that can help you better bear the pain (although they can do that too), they can help lower it.

You can approach this book in a variety of ways. I encourage you to use it in a way that feels best for you. I recommend reading Part One in its entirety, as it will help you understand pain and why drug-free treatments can reduce or relieve your pain: they aren't strategies to simply help you bear or cope with unrelenting pain. As you think about trying new behaviors or adopting new psychological perspectives, start with what feels most relevant or easy to you. Also, understand that you may experience an immediate pain reduction from trying the strategies I review, but that it's likely to take time before your pain reduces significantly or subsides. In my case, it took about three years to see my unrelenting, severe pain move on a scale from a constant 8/10 to intermittent episodes and finally down to a consistent zero. Every person's situation is unique, and thus each chronic pain problem requires its own specific combination of biopsychosocial strategies for securing relief. It can take time to find exactly what that is, so please continue to hold out hope and be patient with yourself. Also, if you have a significant other or caregiver who helps you deal with pain, I encourage them to read this book too. We all need people in our lives who will support us in making the lifestyle changes that we want or need.

Many clients and research volunteers that I've worked with have benefited from the research-backed strategies presented here. You'll read some stories that illustrate how these strategies can be used effectively in real life. These vignettes are composites, combined from the experiences of multiple individuals, to protect confidentiality.

You can start doing much of what you find in this book right away, on your own and/or with the support of a significant other or friends. Additionally, you might read a piece of information that you'd like to discuss further with people on your care team, like your therapist, primary care doctor, or pain specialist. I want to emphasize that if you haven't already, it's vital to have your pain problem evaluated by qualified doctors, and I recommend getting multiple opinions. For example, some physicians will recommend back surgery, whereas others may recommend trying lifestyle changes first. Again, pain is a complex phenomenon impacted by biological, psychological, social, and environmental factors. So your care team should support you in engaging in the strategies you'll read here. You've already started to take charge of your pain by picking up this book. I'm so excited to help you find relief.

YOUR PAIN IS AS UNIQUE AS YOU ARE

As you consider the new skills that you'll learn in this book, stay in communication with your care team. This book will help you create a holistic pain self-management plan. After you've finished reading the book and developed your plan, please share it with care team members and ask for their perspective. Use it to collaborate with them. Don't abandon the recommendations of your health-care providers in favor of something you read here, unless you've thoroughly consulted with them first. This book is chock-full of information, but it does not replace personalized care.

PART ONE

UNDERSTANDING YOUR PAIN

The next three chapters offer up-to-date, science-backed information about chronic pain. Chapter 1 dives into pain neuroscience, which will help you understand how chronic pain works. In Chapters 2 and 3 you'll be invited to reflect on things in your life that might be making your pain better or worse and how you might plan to make changes to support your recovery from chronic pain.

1

Setting the Stage for Healing
Understanding Pain and Your Brain

Believe it or not the pain experience is tied to psychological, emotional, behavioral, and social processes that you can control. Studies suggest that patients who seek out the latest information on the neurophysiology of pain and combine that knowledge with intentional lifestyle changes like physical activity see a reduction in their pain. Known in scientific literature as *pain neuroscience education*, it works primarily by making pain less threatening and by helping people understand on a deeper level how drug-free treatments, which are reviewed in this book, can reduce or eliminate pain. This understanding will be a key support for you as you embark on the difficult task of making lifestyle changes that promote pain relief.

What You Read May Surprise You

What you read in this chapter may surprise you for three interconnected reasons:

1. *Scientists' understanding of chronic pain has undergone rapid changes in recent decades.* Why? Technological advances have contributed to new discoveries and a more sophisticated understanding of pain. For example, neuroimaging techniques, which allow scientists to "see" the

brain and how it works, transformed how we understand and study pain. Functional magnetic resonance imaging, just one of many brain imaging techniques, wasn't discovered until the 1990s. It allows scientists to look at how the brain operates while we're feeling, thinking, or doing certain things (like feeling pain). And it allows observation of how the brain changes in response to pain treatments, including treatment strategies covered in this book. In this chapter, I'll explain some key findings from this research tradition that you can use to help yourself feel better.

2. *The modern neuroscientific understanding of pain is only slowly reaching the public.* Some scientists have estimated that it takes nearly two decades for a scientific finding to be "translated," or regularly offered to patients seeking health care. The "bench-to-bedside" process is complex, but the point remains that it can take a while for science to actually show up in your doctor's office. It's been argued, in fact, that many pain clinicians even lack a modern understanding of how chronic pain works.

3. *Worldwide, there is a shortage of qualified pain psychologists and interdisciplinary pain clinics, which are best equipped to help people understand pain and pursue a holistic pain recovery plan.* Relatedly, insurance companies tend to restrict access to treatments that offer the latest on pain education, such as pain psychology interventions. Primary care physicians also face challenges in getting the training they need to best support patients with pain. Globally, medical school coursework on pain is limited, and many graduates report feeling underprepared to help patients recover from chronic pain. This is obviously a major problem, and repeated calls have been made for curriculum reform, but change is slow. Further, in the United States, physicians are often pressed for time by the demands of insurance companies and might not be able to educate their patients about the complexity of chronic pain, if they do have a good understanding of it, in the time they're allowed to spend with each patient (sometimes as little as 15 minutes). As you move through the health system, it can feel like the only solution to chronic pain is a pill, which can be prescribed quickly in a brief appointment.

This chapter puts current facts about chronic pain directly into your hands. Every day scientists are discovering more and more about chronic pain and its treatment. In this book all I can hope to offer is what is known at the time of this writing. Stay tuned and check the Resources at the back of the book for sources of up-to-date, accurate information on chronic pain treatment.

Pain and Your Brain 101

Let's dive into the modern neuroscientific understanding of chronic pain. In short, we've learned that hypersensitivity of the nervous system—including the brain, spinal cord, and peripheral nerves—is a key reason, if not *the* reason, in several pain conditions, that pain becomes chronic. In comparison with acute injury (such as stepping on a shard of glass or spraining your ankle), chronic pain is less about underlying tissue damage and more about a sensitized nervous system that produces pain in the absence of any real danger. This phenomenon is often compared to an alarm system: pain alerts us to threats, *but it can become faulty*, alerting us to things that aren't dangerous at all. It can even start going off on its own accord. It's as if a leaf were to fall on your car and set off the blaring alarm.

　If you're one of the many people whose pain arose seemingly out of nowhere, perhaps during a stressful time in your life, or one whose pain following an injury or surgery persisted long after your tissues healed, nervous system hypersensitivity may be the primary driver of your pain symptoms. A relatively new term has been coined to describe such conditions: *nociplastic* pain. According to some estimates, most chronic low back pain conditions are primarily nociplastic, with no identifiable tissue damage or problem in the back itself. Also thought to be nociplastic (or significantly so) is chronic pain that

- Emerges during stressful life experiences or in the absence of injury;
- Moves, changes, and spreads throughout the body;
- Gets worse with stress; and/or
- Involves fatigue and sensitivity to light, sound, and smells.

In the case of chronic pain conditions with a genetic basis (sickle cell anemia) or an autoimmune component (rheumatoid arthritis), nervous system hypersensitivity often contributes to pain symptoms and should be targeted in a biopsychosocial pain treatment plan.

Because pain is so attention grabbing, the brain starts to fixate more and more on pain and less and less on pleasurable, safe aspects of our experience, making the pain even worse and all-consuming. Scientists call this phenomenon *reward system dysfunction*. It works like this: we have a limited capacity for attention, so when pain consumes so much of it, the parts of our brain that allow us to pursue and enjoy pleasures, or rewards, start to become faulty and disengaged. If you find that you've lost interest in things you used to love, or that your favorite activities just aren't fun anymore, that's reward system dysfunction at work.

This is a big problem because *rewarding experiences can lower pain*. Positive feelings help your body release pain-relieving and mood-boosting biochemicals, like opioids and serotonin (your body's natural pharmacy)! And when you're feeling curious or interested in something, grateful, content, or confident, it's hard to feel like you're in danger. When you feel safe, your alarm system (your pain alarm) is less likely to go off.

To make matters worse, when you have chronic pain, your brain might not even notice when your pain level goes down a bit. Ordinarily you'd notice at the dentist when the horrible drilling stopped or the painful needle was pulled out of your gums. Without chronic pain in the picture, the reward system registers pain relief as pleasant. But when your reward system glosses over moments of reduced pain, your alarm system stays stuck in high-alert mode. Maybe you can think of a time when you had a lower-than-usual pain day. Instead of feeling relieved or encouraged, maybe you remained stuck in an anxious state, fixated on trying to predict the moment when your pain would ramp up yet again. You weren't able to savor the pain relief or capitalize on it by doing something healthy or fun. *This book will help you rehabilitate your reward system and learn to savor all sorts of rewards again.*

We'll look at this concept in more detail in Chapter 3 but know that positive feelings do more than help pain momentarily. They shift your attention and behavior in ways that help build resilience over the long term. In contrast with negative emotions like anger and sadness, which generally lead to a *narrowing* of attention toward problems and threats, positive feelings *broaden* attention toward a wider range of possibilities. They help you feel more creative and motivated to build what psychology researchers call *resilience resources*, like friendships, new knowledge, hobbies, and habits. These resources, once established, continue to provide you with pain-relieving positive feelings and meaningful experiences.

Here's an example: Maybe you can remember a time when you did something that you used to love before pain started to dominate your life, like when a friend invited you for coffee and your initial reaction was *ugh—I'm really not up for that*. But you went anyway, only to discover that while you were laughing with your friend you didn't even notice your aching back. On your way home, you realized you felt a lot better than when you'd left. And, whether you recognized it at the time or not, this experience deepened your friendship. And so, you nurtured a key ingredient in chronic pain recovery: social support.

Let's tie these concepts back to the car alarm analogy. When your car alarm is going off, you're not appreciating the beautiful blue sky or colorful fall foliage around you. You don't want to stop to enjoy it. You're fixated on the painful sound and frantically search for the button on your fob that silences the noise. The alarm consumes your experience. Although this is completely normal and natural, you miss the opportunity to ease the pain because you can't pay attention to how good it feels to be surrounded by beautiful scenery. You don't experience a positive inspiration to build new healthy habits, like going out in nature each day to enjoy the beauty of autumn. This is reward system dysfunction at work.

If you experience positive feelings only rarely, or struggle to feel motivated to do things that *could* be pleasant, you're in good company. We see evidence of reward system dysfunction across the board in chronic pain. It becomes easy to abandon activities that you once enjoyed, thereby losing access to the internal painkillers (opioids) that we all have, which get released when we experience something as enjoyable. Patients tell me, for example, that things they used to love, like spending time with friends, simply aren't that fun anymore. They describe feeling less and less motivated to see those friends (or do other pleasurable things that might bring relief) because they don't feel like anything helps the pain. They're tired, and nothing feels worthwhile.

I've been there. When my pain was at its worst, I was basically surviving the day in graduate school, taking the bare minimum of classes necessary to stay in my program, and then crashing on the couch in misery. I hardly ever saw any of my fellow classmates. I think many of them started to think I simply didn't like them, especially since I wasn't that open about my health problems.

Nervous system hypersensitivity and reward system dysfunction happen outside of your conscious awareness. Obviously, you aren't trying to make your pain alarm supersensitive! It's like learning how to do something new, such as play the guitar or learn a new dance. As you practice repeatedly the movements start to become effortless because the pathways in your brain that underlie your new skills have gotten more and more efficient. Soon you can do it without even thinking about it. That's how it is with persistent pain: it starts happening automatically.

And now get *this*: that automatic process can be changed. You can reduce nervous system hypersensitivity and improve the brain's reward system functioning with your conscious mind, including engaging in the evidence-based practices presented in this book. Looking back, I really wish I knew about this information when I was grappling with my own chronic pain problem. So please join me in a brief exploration of the neuroscience of pain. I anticipate that you'll come away feeling that you have more control over your pain than you realize.

Pain Is an Alarm System Governed by the Brain

We hate to feel pain, yet it serves a lifesaving purpose. The whole point of pain is to keep us alive by motivating us to escape bodily harm. As I mentioned, pain is like an alarm system—it notifies you that something is amiss and motivates you to act. Tellingly, people with congenital pain insensitivity—a tragic inability to feel pain—rarely survive to adulthood because once they realize they're in danger, it's too late. So it's wonderful to have an alarm system that alerts you to threats. The alarm system doesn't care about your quality of life, however, only your survival. It's better to warn too much than not enough, since ensuring your survival is pain's goal. The brain governs the alarm system: *100 percent of the time pain is produced by the brain*. If your brain thinks that you might be in danger, somewhere, somehow, it will produce pain, even if you're made miserable in the process. Pain doesn't care if you miss your kid's soccer game because of a pounding headache, only that you keep on living.

If this information comes as a surprise, understand that pain, including chronic pain, was historically conceptualized in the Western medical system as caused by underlying tissue damage and solved by curing that damage. This idea is part of the biomedical model of health, which claims that if you have a physical complaint, it must be because something has physically gone awry that demands correction through medicines or procedures. Dr. Emeran Mayer argues in his book *The Mind-Gut Connection* that traditionally, Western medicine has viewed the body as a mechanical device like a car with complex parts. The physician is like an auto mechanic who fixes a single broken piece of that device with surgery or pills. Although this model supports a lucrative health-care industry with expensive pharmaceuticals and procedures, it fails to help our society achieve good health, and it particularly fails people with chronic pain and illness.

The biomedical model is flawed, but it does apply somewhat to acute pain. The pain you feel after spraining your ankle motivates you to rest; after your tissues have healed, the pain vanishes. But the model fails to explain chronic pain; for many people pain persists long after injuries have healed. And even with acute pain it's the brain that makes the final decision on the extent to which you experience pain.

A few striking examples illustrate that it's not tissue damage or dysfunction that produces pain, but rather the brain. The first is phantom limb pain in amputees, where pain is felt in limbs that aren't there at all. Another is an often-cited case described in *The British Medical Journal* involving a construction worker who stepped on a nail that pierced through his boot through to the other side. In excruciating pain he headed for the emergency department of a nearby hospital, where he was given opioids for pain control. His doctors then removed the boot only to see that the nail had passed between his toes, his foot unscathed. This man's brain made a calculation that it was beneficial to his survival to produce pain based on visual input that suggested potential bodily harm. *Obviously no one-to-one relationship between tissue damage and pain exists.*

The lack of direct association between tissue abnormalities and chronic pain has been known for quite a while. For instance, a group of pain researchers in the 1990s scanned the backs of people with and without chronic low back pain with magnetic resonance imaging and found a similar frequency of disc abnormalities in both groups. So often patients with chronic low back pain are told that their pain is caused by "slipped discs," "herniated discs," and the like. Yet we all demonstrate degeneration in the spine as we age, and only some of us have chronic low back pain. Similarly, in knee osteoarthritis, the extent of joint degeneration is only moderately associated with how much pain people report, and in up to a third of patients, knee replacement surgery doesn't cure their knee pain. These findings suggest that a key mechanism of chronic pain is a hypersensitive nervous system, with the brain at the helm.

Remarkable cases of people reporting little to no pain despite real danger also show us that the brain produces pain. For example, as reported by anesthesiologist Dr. Henry Beecher, during World War II soldiers undergoing surgery following battle wounds said they had significantly less pain than civilians undergoing the same kinds of procedures. The meaning assigned to the situation might have been paramount in determining the pain experience: the soldiers viewed their injury and associated surgery as a ticket to safety (being shipped home), whereas civilians felt that surgery was an interruption of normal life, rife with uncertainty, potential complications, and a lengthy recovery. Again, the brain's calculus ultimately hinges on whether it thinks life and limb are at stake. Multiple studies now show that our thoughts (such as the meaning we give to our state of health) are one input that the brain uses to make this calculation. We'll talk more about the brain's decision-making process and how we can influence it through our conscious thoughts and behaviors in the next section.

You might wonder, what about the nerves in our arms, legs, and organs? Don't they communicate pain? In fact, we don't have nerves in our body that definitively signal "pain." We have nerves known as *nociceptors* that pain neuroscience educators aptly call "danger receptors" because they notify us that something's weighing on us too heavily, something's too hot, or we're in contact with a dangerous substance, for instance. But impulses traveling from these nerves to the brain are not necessary for us to experience pain, as the construction worker example shows. Nor are they sufficient for pain, as shown by the injured soldiers example. The brain ultimately decides whether pain is appropriate.

You may not feel the need right now to take an even deeper dive into pain neurophysiology, but to get the most out of recent advances in our understanding of chronic pain it's useful to know something about the brain's decision-making process. First, how does it decide to trigger the alarm?

How the Brain Sets Off the Alarm

Let's go back to the construction worker who was in agony after stepping on a nail that he thought had gone all the way through his foot. The man's visual experiences and beliefs were key messages that the brain incorporated into its decision to send the danger signal we call pain. But, as this example shows, the brain does not have access to an "objective" picture of reality. Rather, the brain must constantly sort through a staggering amount of ambiguous sensory and perceptual information, coming from inside and outside the body, and make guesses about our state of health and safety based on that information. It also draws heavily on prior experiences about health and safety in its guesswork. For example, adverse childhood experiences like trauma or growing up with affectionless, overprotective parents are associated with a greater risk of developing a chronic pain condition later on in life.

After the brain makes its best guess, it orchestrates pain and related physiological responses (inflammation, stress hormones, and so forth) accordingly in an effort to keep us alive and well. So for the construction worker, all it may have taken for the brain to flip on the pain switch was the shocking visual picture of a big nail sticking up out of his boot—of course it must have gone through his foot, an understandable but inaccurate assumption. On the other hand this worker may also have had a history of stepping on sharp objects lodged firmly in his memory. Or he may have had parents who curtailed his childhood adventures based on exaggerated risks to their son.

The factors that play a role in the brain's decision to create a painful danger warning are complicated. Let's say you're at the beach with friends, enjoying a bonfire and barbecue. Suddenly, you step on a shard of glass. To decide whether producing pain will benefit your survival, the brain will process signals coming from the nerves in your foot along with many other inputs: psychological factors (maybe you're worried about how deeply you've been cut or your risk of infection), social processes (the fact that friends are there to support you), emotions (such as fear), prior learning (such as that sharp glass tends to be dangerous), and environmental features (how far are you from the nearest hospital?). If the answer is yes, *whammo*, you experience pain and become motivated to remove the shard of glass, get help from others, and stay off your foot until your tissues have healed.

Pain Involves More than Biology

This is the contemporary, neuroscientific understanding of pain. Rather than a biomedical phenomenon (a direct relationship between tissue damage and pain), it's a biopsychosocial one, with the brain making a final decision on whether pain is appropriate by considering social, psychological, biological, environmental, and emotional information. This biopsychosocial model of pain is the prevailing model guiding chronic pain research at present.

Because Western medicine has been so firmly rooted in the biomedical model, it may seem hard to believe that psychological and social factors can substantially exacerbate pain. It may be even more incredible to think these factors can also *relieve* pain! Yet we've all had experiences that illustrate how powerfully our thoughts, attention, and context impact the level of pain we do (or don't) experience. Think about sports. Say you're playing soccer with friends, and the competition is fierce. You're so focused on winning and enjoying the match that it's only afterward that you notice your calf is bleeding. In the heat of competition, you felt no pain at all!

As you can probably sense already, we can impact the brain's guesswork through our own conscious thoughts and behaviors. It's not as if pain is some objective reality over which we have no control. Our feelings, thoughts, actions, and environments are all different types of inputs to the brain that we can consciously alter for our brain's benefit. In essence there are thoughts, behaviors, and environments that communicate safety and well-being to the brain, which are liable to reduce pain. On the other hand, there are thoughts, behaviors, and environments that communicate threat and danger to our nervous system, which promote pain. Furthermore, we can retrain the brain away from a narrowed, fixated attention to pain and toward a broadened perspective with the ability to notice, savor, and enjoy natural rewards. We can "rehabilitate" our brain's reward system, in turn reducing pain.

*Neuroplasticity: Getting Good at Sounding the Alarm
at the Expense of Joy and Well-Being*

As noted earlier the more the nervous system produces pain, the better
it gets at producing it. This capacity is known as *neuroplasticity*, or the
brain's ability to change in structure and function. Neuroplasticity can
be a great thing. For instance, the more we play a sport, the better we
get at it and the more automatic it becomes—we can perform skilled
motor movements without even thinking about them. The more people
practice meditation the better they get at being in the present, and we
see corresponding changes in brain circuits that underlie attention and
concentration.

In the case of chronic pain, unfortunately, neuroplasticity is unhelpful. Pain physiologists Lorimer Moseley and David Butler compare the
brain to an orchestra that's been practicing a "pain tune" so much that
it knows how to play it loud, fast, and constantly and now can't remember how to play anything else. Neuroplasticity can lead to all kinds of
hypersensitivity common in chronic pain conditions: feeling more pain
in response to things that used to cause less pain; feeling discomfort in
response to harmless stimuli, like a tag on your shirt; and feeling pain
that spreads beyond the site of the initial injury. The brain gets so good
at alerting us to threats that it even becomes concerned about sensations
from our own bodies that are completely harmless. Everyone experiences
natural fluctuations in bodily sensations: feelings of pressure, warmth,
etc. People living with chronic pain are much more likely to interpret
these sensations as threatening or painful because their brain is on high
alert to identify dangers.

More Pain and Less Pleasure

Let's come back to the pain tune. Beyond upping your pain, it can dis-
rupt the brain's reward system, making it difficult to look forward to and
enjoy pleasurable, rewarding, and meaningful aspects of your life. A critical overture that the brain forgets how to play is the one about joy, pleasure, and meaning. We need that overture not only for happiness but,
critically, for pain management. Research resoundingly shows that positive feelings and activities have natural pain-relieving effects. Yet under
chronic pain conditions, thanks to neuroplasticity, we can't access them

as easily. The brain has finite attentional resources, and much of them are being sapped by pain—how it feels, what it means, how to fix it. Resources are becoming less available to seek out and notice pleasurable, rewarding experiences, or even neutral, nonthreatening experiences. This is not your fault, of course. Pain is attention grabbing by its nature. And the distressing thoughts (how long will it last?) and feelings (fear, sadness, anger) that surround it start to win out. However, it's possible to retrain the brain to experience more joy and pleasure and seek out environments that promote positive feelings of safety, joy, and well-being.

Turning Neuroplasticity into an Ally

Importantly, you can retrain the brain while the alarm bell is going off. It's easy to feel like you need to wait for pain to get better to be able to experience joy and pleasure again. Commonly (and understandably), people feel they need pain-relieving medication or intervention (surgery, injection) before feeling safe enough to go out and do things like hiking, walking, having dinner out with friends, or taking an art class. It's easy to postpone your life and let pain take center stage. This way of responding is natural. Remember that acute pain is designed to get us to move out of harm's way and then rest until our damaged tissues have healed. But resting and avoiding activities after pain has become chronic while waiting around for an effective drug or surgery isn't what's needed. Although your pain seems to scream at you to rest, withdraw, become afraid or angry, and shove fun things to the side until the pain sensation itself is lowered, you must consciously override these impulses and find ways to engage in and savor activities that you like and value. This in and of itself *is* a treatment. It will help your brain learn that it doesn't need to continue to keep creating a pain experience as well as release the body's natural painkillers (opioids).

Because of neuroplasticity, you can retrain your brain to notice rewards and pleasures once again. In upcoming chapters you'll learn strategies to get your brain and body out of high-alert mode and into a state of greater balance, ease, happiness, and well-being. Please know that it will likely take time and dedicated practice for your brain to unlearn what it has learned, but you might also notice an immediate benefit from using the strategies in this book. And you're not embarking on an exhausting, max-intensity, lifelong mental training program. Retraining your brain and changing behaviors is like weight training or learning to ride a bike: it's hard to build initial muscle mass, but less effort is required to maintain the muscle that you've built. Bike riding takes all your attention at first but then becomes automatic. As you start experiencing pain relief from the strategies you'll learn, you'll likely settle on a combination of practices that work best for you, and that will help maintain the gains you've made.

The Role of Inflammation

Inflammation, the body's natural response to harmful stimuli, is a vital part of its alarm system. After injury your body releases various chemicals and molecules that fight infection and promote tissue healing. So in acute pain situations inflammation is a good thing because it's needed for tissue repair. When you see redness and swelling after spraining your ankle or having your wisdom teeth pulled, that's inflammation. The swollen area becomes tender to the touch because inflammatory chemicals stimulate danger receptors (nociceptors) both at the site of the injury and near it. Your alarm system *really* wants you to notice the injury as well as protect an area as large as possible from further damage. The brain is very responsive to inflammatory chemicals, and when it detects them, it is quick to construct a pain experience. Scientifically, the causal link between inflammation and pain is robust (they don't simply correlate or happen at the same time). To demonstrate this, scientists have experimented by injecting people with inflammation-inducing bacteria (with their consent of course!) to observe its effects. They found that increased inflammation, heightened bodily pain, and increased negative mood tended to result more than when something benign, like a saline injection, was given.

   Unlike acute injury situations, chronically elevated inflammation is not a good thing and contributes directly to ongoing pain. It's another way in which your alarm system can get stuck in crisis mode. Like chronic versus acute pain, chronic inflammation loses its protective function. Rheumatoid arthritis, complex regional pain syndrome, diabetic neuropathic pain, chronic widespread pain, fibromyalgia, chronic low back pain, and temporomandibular disorder are just a few examples of chronic pain conditions with elevated systemic inflammation relative to healthy conditions. Interestingly, whole-body, systemic inflammation has been documented in conditions where pain is felt only in one area of the body (like the lower back or jaw). Systemic inflammation also contributes to fatigue and cognitive issues, which often accompany chronic pain, as well as mental health conditions like anxiety and depression that worsen pain.

If you've been living with chronic pain, even if it's isolated, it's very possible that elevated inflammation is playing a role in your symptoms. Again, your body's alarm system, which includes inflammation, is overreacting. It's faulty. But I have some fantastic news: you can lower your level of inflammation, which will in turn lower your pain. Science shows that an anti-inflammatory diet, physical activity, and improved sleep can have especially positive effects on inflammation and therefore pain. We'll dive into that in greater depth in Part Four.

I bet you've heard it a million times before, but I promise you, science has given us new and exciting insights into how and why these lifestyle habits lower pain and that their effects can be extraordinary. I experienced some of the biggest reductions in my pain by strictly following an anti-inflammatory diet for 90 days on the advice of one of my physicians. It was tough, but I was desperate, and in the end the results were phenomenal. To this day I maintain that diet as best I can to help keep migraines, shoulder pain, and neck pain at bay. It's also worth noting that pain self-management strategies (think anything that you can control and don't rely on a doctor for, like meditation, relaxation training, or getting social support) have the potential to reduce inflammation by lessening the fight-or-flight response. Studies have shown that pain management strategies like mindfulness-based practices, stress reduction techniques, and behavioral activation (increasing engagement in valued pursuits) can lower inflammation.

Expectations Matter

Because the brain lacks a complete picture of reality, it has to fill in the gaps. Fascinating new research indicates that the brain wants our experiences to match its predictions. For example, if the brain expects the body to heal (if we enter a healing environment with medical rituals, or we develop a mindset that we are on a path toward healing, for example), it will begin to interpret bodily sensations in accord with that prediction, nudging us toward health. Research illustrates this quite dramatically: chronic pain patients who take placebo (sugar) pills over a period of weeks and are openly told by the research staff that they don't contain active ingredients, report significant improvements in symptoms!

Researchers conducting these trials theorize that subconsciously the brain is getting health and safety signals from the simple act of taking a pill, and it then interprets what's happening in the body in a manner consistent with those signals. Laboratory studies have shown that people perceive more pain in response to a potentially harmful stimulus (like heat) when they are simultaneously exposed to a danger signal (such as a red light) versus a safety signal (like a blue light). Our world has conditioned us to associate the color red with heat and danger and the color blue with coolness and safety. Findings like these illustrate that prior expectations and beliefs are part of the brain's process of guessing how threatened or safe we are. Worldwide, studies confirm that expectations and beliefs shape our pain experience. Conversely, if the brain forms a prediction that we are sick and only getting worse, it will interpret bodily sensations as threatening, making pain more likely.

As we close this chapter, take a moment to consider what conscious expectations you hold about your pain journey. Do you expect, even in a small way, that your pain can be reduced or eliminated? If so, take a moment to notice and appreciate this positive expectation. On the other hand, do you have expectations that you'll never improve? Can you question or challenge these expectations?

FOR MORE INFORMATION
ON PAIN NEUROSCIENCE EDUCATION

When you're ready to take a deeper dive into pain neurophysiology, you can seek out the many volumes that have been written for the public explaining how and why the brain makes the final decision on whether we experience pain. Notable among these is pain physiologists Dr.

David Butler and Lorimer Moseley's *Explain Pain* (*www.noigroup.com/ product/explain-pain-second-edition*) series. Further, there is a relatively new evidence-based smartphone app called Curable (*www.curablehealth.com*) that can help you deepen your understanding of pain neuroscience and apply it to your own situation. Lin Health (*https://lin.health*) is another online program grounded in modern pain neuroscience. The most exciting thing about pain neuroscience education is that it shows us that we have more control over pain than was once believed.

2

Identifying Threats

C hronic pain is like a foreign language—it may be telling you something important, but at first, it's hard to understand. It can be your body's way of letting you know that there's some problem in your life like you're overworked, overly stressed, physically inactive, or experiencing family conflict. The key is to figure out your body's language and what you can learn from it. I love this metaphor because, as discussed in Chapter 1, the chronic pain brain is on high alert, constantly scanning for threats and interpreting innocuous information as potential danger. So a good starting point is to take inventory of the possible threats in your life, small and large, and consider if and how they may be contributing to your pain problem. Next, identify which threats you can control and reduce, even in a small way. Threats can be psychological, emotional, and social as well as physical. As I described in the Introduction, although there were biological influences on my pain problem, it became life-interfering only when I encountered relational threats that were too much to bear.

In Chapter 1 I suggested that each person has a unique set of "ingredients" that will help them recover from chronic pain. Some ingredients consist of relatively small changes that you can easily add to your pain recovery recipe. Michael was a dedicated social justice advocate who struggled with chronic pain. He came to realize that checking the news on his smartphone multiple times a day was exposing his brain to threatening information relentlessly. One piece of his holistic pain self-management plan was taking regular "vacations" from the news. He easily stayed abreast of important news events while reducing unnecessary danger messages to his nervous system. While taking this step didn't magically make Michael's pain go away, he noticed an immediate reduction in worry and anxiety. Anxious worry can ramp up pain, so this was a key step forward for him. Michael's story is an example that shows how some threats in your life might be easily addressed with simple changes in behavior. Other threats may take more time and effort to manage. For now, simply reflect and, with an open mind, consider the information in this chapter and how it might apply to you.

In this chapter you'll learn about common threats that have been shown to adversely impact pain directly and/or indirectly through increased stress. Stress is defined as the perception that we lack the resources to deal with what's happening in our environment. This can be scary, so our threat-surveillance system activates.

The list of threats that follow may not be exhaustive, since new research is emerging every day, but it includes what I see as the most impactful threats identified in the scientific literature on pain, fear, and well-being. As you read about these risk factors and reflect on their role in your own chronic pain, picture your capacity to manage threats as if they exist in a bucket. Even though your bucket is large, at a certain point it will overflow, and symptoms will appear. So any potential threat is worth addressing.

But also keep in mind that risk factors can interact and overlap with one another as well as cumulatively impact pain. This means that addressing one threat might also favorably impact other, related threats while reducing your cumulative total. It also means that progress might not necessarily be linear. At times you might feel like you're taking a few steps forward, only to take a few steps back. You can think of healing as a spiral rather than a straight line: sometimes you're going up, and sometimes you're going down, but you're always tracking toward the center.

Finally, you can also think of your efforts to adopt new strategies as setting an *upward spiral* motion. You may have heard about downward spirals (injury leading to pain leading to depression), but upward spirals (a friendship leading to increased social activity leading to reduced pain) are equally possible.

Trauma

Untreated early life or recent traumas can sensitize the nervous system and make it hypervigilant to threats. Traumas are events that make us feel unsafe, that threaten our very existence. They include "Big T" traumas like physical abuse and neglect, medical traumas, or natural disasters as well as accumulated "Little T" traumas like emotional invalidation, criticism, or being ignored in early child-caregiver relationships.

When you've experienced trauma of any sort, your brain wants to be sure that you don't experience it or anything like it again. So it enthusiastically kicks up the intensity of its threat-surveillance system. Trauma history is far more prevalent in people with chronic pain than in pain-free people. Prior trauma has been associated with a two- to three-fold increase in the likelihood of developing a chronic pain or fatigue disorder characterized by nervous system hypersensitivity, like fibromyalgia, chronic widespread pain, irritable bowel syndrome, temporomandibular disorder, and chronic fatigue syndrome. These findings speak to the nervous system hypersensitivity that can emerge in the wake of trauma.

If you've experienced trauma, you can benefit from biopsychosocial pain treatment (that is, using the strategies offered in this book) to the same degree as people who don't have a trauma history. You'll find more on how to address trauma in Chapter 5.

REFLECT: For now, simply think about these questions: Have you experienced trauma? Is it possible that the effects of trauma are playing a role in your current physical and emotional health?

Untreated Mental Health Conditions

Anxiety and depression are common conditions that make pain worse and make it harder to stay engaged in valued life activities like work, school, or social activities. Anxiety involves excessive fear and worry about imagined future events and physiological hyperarousal (think rapid, shallow breathing, sweaty palms, and digestive issues), while depression involves low motivation, little interest or pleasure in doing things you once enjoyed, and feelings of hopelessness. It can also involve thoughts of hurting yourself. Depression and chronic pain very frequently occur together and may share some of the same underlying pathophysiological mechanisms, namely inflammation and reward system dysfunction. So, by treating one you can potentially improve both conditions.

REFLECT: Has your mental health deteriorated because of chronic pain? Have other people in your life encouraged you to make changes to support your mental health, like get into counseling? While mental health conditions like anxiety and depression need to be diagnosed by a mental health professional, you can take this moment to reflect on your mental health.

If you're ever in crisis and need to speak with a counselor immediately, dial 988.

Self-Criticism

Many of us, most of the time, would never talk to a friend the way we do to ourselves. Sadly, self-aversion is ubiquitous in our society. I've honestly never had a therapy client who didn't add a layer of self-judgment to their raw experience, be it feelings of fear, the loss of a relationship, obsessive thinking patterns, a chronic health condition . . . the list goes on. The joys and sorrows of life present themselves, and rather than encouraging ourselves with kindness and understanding through it all, we go to war internally. We lose a job, something falls through the cracks, we don't show up authentically in relationships the way we'd like, we say things we regret, we have a hard time dealing with difficult people in our lives; in other words, we act like human beings. But we add the thought *I'm bad doing or being like this. I'm falling short. I should be better.* The inner critic is mean and threatening and puts us into a state of high alert and negativity. Self-criticism leads to feelings of shame, tension, and anger at oneself. Research repeatedly shows, in diverse research designs, populations, and laboratories, that negative emotions like these make physical pain worse.

If you're struggling with self-criticism, it's not your fault. We learn to dislike ourselves by various routes. Early childhood experience is a big one. As humans we have a long and vulnerable childhood in which the brain is under construction, and we learn templates for relating to ourselves and others that follow us into adulthood. You may have had early life caregivers (teachers, parents, babysitters) who neglected, criticized, shamed, or acted violently toward you when you were in distress, behaving in ways that were inconvenient, or falling short of a particular standard. Developmentally, children have a limited ability to see the world through perspectives other than their own; so they erroneously interpret aggressive (yelling or worse), withdrawing (ignoring, abandoning), or otherwise dysfunctional behavior from adults as their own fault rather than due to larger forces (such as unhealed intergenerational patterns or wounds, trauma, societal violence, a lack of parental supports, or social inequities impacting the family). If you felt unsafe in relationships with your early caregivers, you may have had thoughts like, *I must be bad for my caregiver to act this way. I need to change how I am to make sure my caregiver will protect me in a world I can't navigate on my own. Rather than wild, free, and real, I should be perfect.* Buddhist peace activist and poet Thich Nhat Hanh writes that as children, we're naturally sensitive and wanting of love, such that even one harsh word from an adult can really hurt. No matter how safe or traumatic our early experience was, we all have an inner child that needs to be heard, cared for, and loved. We'll dive into self-compassion as an inner healing strategy in Chapter 8. You can reparent your inner child by listening to it and offering it kindness, understanding, and love.

Of course, we receive messages that we're not OK from countless sources beyond our early life caregivers or immediate family. Friends, peers, romantic partners, and others might reject certain things about us, and we jump to try to change ourselves to avoid abandonment. The dominant culture in the United States is one that places a premium on production and consumption. Our inherent worth, beauty, and goodness get lost in a toxic system where our worth is equated with how hard we work and how busy we are. We get cut off from the natural world to which we belong, and we forget how to slow down. We're told that if we don't belong to the dominant social group (White, cisgender, ablebodied, male, Christian, and heterosexual, and if you do happen to be male, you're not allowed to cry), there's something wrong with us.

REFLECT: How loud is your inner critic? Would learning how to love yourself exactly as you are help calm your nervous system?

Chronic Pain Stigma

Chronic pain status is a socially stigmatized identity. Having pain that doesn't abate, and particularly a type of pain for which no underlying biomedical cause can be identified, is a violation of what Western society teaches us about it: that it is something that reflects an acute injury that then eventually goes away. The social stigma around chronic pain causes emotional distress (negative emotions), which worsens pain.

If you feel like society has rejected and marginalized you because of your pain, it's not "all in your head"; research has shown that people with chronic pain report more experiences of discrimination in daily life than people without it. Patients tell me they wonder if they're defective in some way because their pain isn't improving and the pain-free people around them just don't get it or, worse, doubt whether they're telling the truth about their pain. You might feel like you constantly need to prove to others that you're in pain because they can't see the pain and they don't believe you. Maybe you've felt like you were being labeled, implicitly or explicitly, as a "difficult patient," "demanding," or "an addict." Maybe you've had people say to you dismissively, "Just learn to live with it" or look at you accusingly when using an accessible parking space. You're not alone. Trust that your experience is valid and real and that you are an incredible human being worthy of love and protection.

REFLECT: Have you been internalizing the stigmatizing messages that society spreads about people living with chronic pain, such as that you're weak, a burden, or psychologically unwell?

Pain-Related Worry

When you have chronic pain, it's only natural to worry about it. *How long will it last? Is there something wrong with my body that the doctors aren't catching? What if I never get better? I want to go to that movie with friends, but how much worse will my pain get? Maybe I should stay home. Everyone says I need to move more to ultimately feel better, but I'm so scared I'll hurt myself. What if my pain gets worse and I can't make it through the workday?* And on, and on, and on.

Your mind wants to protect you, so it will envision every kind of catastrophe and encourage you to think through how you'll deal with it. Ruminating about pain, letting it take up an enormous amount of space in your mind, and doubting that you can cope effectively with it are mental threats that keep your physiology in high-alert mode. There are the pain sensations themselves, and then there is all the mental proliferation that goes on about those sensations that can ultimately make them worse. Remember that the goal is to help your brain learn that you're safe, that you're not in peril. When you ruminate about imagined scary outcomes, you're essentially telling your brain that yes, you are under threat. Keep producing pain, brain. Fortunately, researchers have developed tools to help people reduce how much they worry about pain, and studies show that these tools can reduce pain severity. In Part Two, you'll learn how to lower pain-related worry to help yourself feel better.

REFLECT: How much chronic worry about pain (and perhaps other things as well) may be contributing to your overall threat level?

Discrimination

Discrimination, based on one or more devalued social identities, is a source of ongoing traumatic stress that can worsen pain. Among the social identity constructs that may be associated with chronic pain risk, pain researchers have most frequently investigated Black race and female gender.

Research studies show that Black patients often report greater nervous system (pain) hypersensitivity than White patients, which is not surprising given the multiple levels of discrimination and threat that Black individuals in America face on a daily basis in addition to the ancestral trauma of slavery. The construct of "race" itself is not a risk factor for pain; rather, discrimination is threatening and can put the danger alarm on high alert.

Similar findings emerge for women, who commonly report higher pain than men. Women are often stereotyped as overreacting to diseases or being emotionally hypersensitive and willing to voice their struggles with pain, which has an obvious parallel to the female hysteria diagnosis of antiquity. Scientific data show that women face discrimination, and the psychological distress caused by that discrimination can sensitize the pain alarm. For instance, experimental data have shown that women perceive more pain and show greater brain activation in regions that process pain while they view images depicting gender-based discrimination relative to neutral images. Let's extrapolate this to the real world with an example. Picture a woman who lives with chronic pain. She is passed up for a promotion in favor of a male colleague with significantly less experience at the organization. The injustice of it causes stress, disappointment, and frustration, not to mention real financial consequences for her family. Consequently, her pain ramps up.

Discrimination can cause pain. Our threat surveillance (pain) system detects the threat and wants to protect us, so it sets off the alarm more easily.

What can you do about discrimination? The threat of discrimination will of course never be eliminated until structural inequities no longer exist. In the meantime, you must shore up supports to stay well in the face of the social discrimination that targets your unique combination of social identities, including chronic pain status. I'll talk more about how to help your brain feel safer and increase your well-being despite social discriminatory threats in Parts Two and Three, and in Chapter 5 on addressing trauma.

REFLECT: For now, simply think about discrimination as a source of psychological distress that may be worsening your pain and recognize that you have the power to strengthen sources of protection, safety, and joy in the face of these influences.

Physical Inactivity

The body is designed to be in motion regularly throughout the day. As pain physiologists Lorimer Moseley and David Butler describe in *Explain Pain*, the brain perceives a lack of movement as a threat. Acid and other by-products build up in the tissues when we sit still for too long and activate our danger receptors (nociceptors). The brain receives that information and becomes more likely to produce pain. Physical activity also promotes healthy blood circulation, which delivers nutrients and oxygen to the tissues.

Physical inactivity is often caused by a fear of movement, technically known as *kinesiophobia*. People with pain often fear that if they move, they'll cause further injury or a flare-up of symptoms. Listening to the fear, they move very little or not at all. Deconditioning, defined as a significant reduction in muscle strength and cardiovascular fitness, can set in, which makes it harder to participate in social, work, or volunteer opportunities. Missing out on important life events and activities worsens pain, physical functioning, and well-being in a vicious cycle.

REFLECT: Is physical inactivity a potential threat? You must override the impulse to remain still to protect your body. You *can* increase activity in ways that feel manageable and safe. I'll talk about how to do that in Part Four.

Insomnia

Poor sleep increases the activity of the sympathetic nervous system, a branch of the nervous system that helps us fight, flee, or freeze in the face of threats. It also increases inflammation and lowers our ability to experience positive feelings in the daytime. Thus it's a triple threat for pain. Many people with chronic pain suffer from insomnia. It's not just that chronic pain makes it hard to sleep, research compellingly shows that poor sleep causes pain. For example, during overnight laboratory visits, researchers will study people, waking them up all night long, and then, the next day, test the sensitivity of their pain alarms, inflammation levels, and emotional states. It's not a pretty picture. Pain and inflammation increase while emotional health decreases. There are drug-free interventions for insomnia that work for people with chronic pain, which are discussed in Part Four.

REFLECT: Are you getting about eight hours of good sleep a night? Do you feel rested after you sleep? If you slept better, could you be doing better? Do you want to direct some energy toward building healthy sleep habits? Stay tuned for helpful information in Part Four.

Poor Diet

The body is designed to receive a diversity of nutrients from foods, which we get by "eating the rainbow," a variety of vegetables and fruits. However, the presence of harmful chemicals in our food and the absence of nutrients is threatening and can ramp up the body's alarm system. Food additives (think things on a food label that you can't pronounce, like titanium dioxide, monosodium glutamate, polysorbate 80, or butylated hydroxyanisole) are frequently added to processed meats and packaged foods to make them look better and have a longer shelf life. Although these sorts of additives are not good for your health, there is no law against their use in the United States.

Research indicates that food additives can increase inflammation (again, inflammation increases pain). Remember that inflammation is designed to attack and eliminate threats entering the body, such as bacteria. The body reacts similarly to the junk we're eating from packaged food. The standard American diet consisting of sugary foods, refined grains (like white bread), processed meats (cured bacon, sausage, chicken nuggets), and low fruit/vegetable intake sensitizes danger receptors by causing excessive inflammation. It's a threat to our physiology.

REFLECT: Consider the role of diet as it relates to your condition. Are you eating a lot of processed foods? Are you eating the rainbow? Are you eating a lot of meat and few fruits and vegetables? Has anyone on your care team helped you develop a personalized nutrition plan to reduce your pain? Have you stuck to that plan faithfully for at least a few months?

Smartphone and Social Media Overuse

Smartphones have basically taken control of our lives. They are addictive by design, and as a society we've taken the bait. Constant access to the internet (news, social media sites), email, calendars and to-do lists, interruptive sounds, blue light . . . the list goes on, exposes our brains to diverse sources of threatening information, nonstop. Sure, it's important to stay connected and abreast of current events yet grabbing for our phones mindlessly and frequently exposes us to all kinds of scary events and possibilities and makes us think that such things are *likely* to happen to us too. Searching the internet for health-related information exposes us to a wide variety of scary and tragic stories of suffering and disease. Our brains aren't designed for this. We didn't evolve as a species with smartphones or social media—the stimulation is overwhelming and makes us fearful and tense. Worse, internet scrolling takes us away from sources of true, sustainable joy and meaning like friendships, the natural world, and creative pursuits. Phone use promotes physical inactivity and might even contribute to neck pain through excessive strain and tension in the neck muscles.

REFLECT: When you pick up your phone, what are you really longing for? Peace, ease, joy, a break? To feel loved or safe? Pain relief? Is your phone really giving you those things? What do you lose by going online?

Job-Related Stressors

Research suggests that job stressors are associated with pain and could even be a precursor for it. Interpersonal conflict, being asked to work too much, and having little control or autonomy in the workplace have been shown to be predictors of stress-related physical symptoms including pain, sleep disturbance, fatigue, appetite loss, and others. If you feel trapped, threatened, or drained by your work environment, your job situation could be ramping up your nervous system.

REFLECT: Do you work in an environment that feels safe and supportive? Do you have a sense of control over what goes on during your day? Do you have positive and fulfilling relationships with coworkers? Are you being asked to complete a reasonable (not excessive) number of tasks on a given day? Are you encouraged to have work-life balance? If the answer to any or all these questions is no, it's possible that work-related stressors are threatening your nervous system and contributing to your pain.

Relationship Problems

If there's one factor that resoundingly emerges as beneficial for health, including pain, it's the presence of gratifying and supportive social relationships. Research shows that negative and hostile social interactions, as well as loneliness, exacerbate pain. As a species group dynamics ensured our survival; we can't do life alone. Social networks are so key to our survival that having them break down is extremely threatening. Yet maintaining high-quality relationships that are safe, rewarding, and fulfilling is one of our greatest challenges.

A wide variety of relationship situations could threaten your well-being and sensitize your alarm system. Maybe you spend a lot of time alone due to an absence of fulfilling friendships or familial relationships. If you're like most people I know, you might find yourself struggling to be authentic with others and putting on a mask to try to be liked. Maybe you're on the receiving end of emotionally abusive tactics like criticism, shaming, or blaming, or perhaps your partner is struggling to get help with a substance use disorder that detracts from your ability to connect authentically. Maybe you struggle to set boundaries with others (saying yes when you really mean no), and you're exhausted; or maybe you notice yourself lashing out in anger toward others when you're hurting inside.

If you feel like your needs for connection aren't being met, for whatever collection of reasons unique to you, I highly encourage you to do what you can to improve your social well-being with the help of the information you'll find in Chapter 6. The "social" component of the biopsychosocial model of pain has received less attention than the psychological and biological, which is unfortunate because pain unfolds within the social world. Relationship stressors can be an intense source of distress, while good relationships are an enduring source of joy and happiness.

REFLECT: Take a moment to take stock of your social situation. Do you feel safe and connected with other people in your life? You'll find more about improving relationships and how significant others in your life can best help you lower your pain in Chapter 6.

EXERCISE

Which of the threats described in this chapter are most applicable to you? Which feel important to work on, and which do you feel like you already have under control? Are there any threats that you feel are important for you that weren't mentioned? Write in the spaces below or in a journal whatever thoughts, feelings, or reactions come up without censoring yourself, and/or use the checklist that follows.

....

....

....

My Risk Factors

Check off each risk that applies to you.

❑ Trauma

❑ Untreated mental health conditions

❑ Self-criticism

❑ Chronic pain stigma

❑ Pain-related worry

❑ Discrimination

❑ Physical inactivity

❑ Insomnia

❑ Poor diet

❑ Smartphone and social media overuse

❑ Job-related stressors

❑ Relationship problems

❑ Others (write or reflect on any others that come to mind for you in this
   section)

....

....

....

3

Identifying Sources of Joy and Meaning

In Chapter 2 you learned about sources of threats that may be ramping up your nervous system. This chapter delves into how positive emotions can help get you out of pain. I'll help you identify and build on sources of joy and meaning already present in your life (which may have fallen by the wayside due to pain) and review science-backed sources of joy and happiness that may be worth considering.

Why do we have positive emotions? Why do we do things that are meaningful to us and that provide us opportunities to experience joy? The conventional wisdom used to be that positive feelings are a *result* of having close friends, good health, enough money, and doing things that are fun and meaningful. But more recent research studies indicate that when we feel good, we think and act in more expansive, creative, and health-benefiting ways that in turn build supportive, life-affirming resources that endure. In other words, positive emotions *lead* us to do things that are good for ourselves and others. For example, when you feel happy and at ease, you're more likely to invite a friend out for coffee; that friend is then likely to reciprocate in some way, perhaps by inviting you out to dinner or helping you out in a time of need. The formation of an enduring friendship bond is set into motion. When you're feeling energized and interested, you're more likely to do something creative (say a gardening project), which keeps your mind sharp and your body active, thus promoting longevity. But how are positive emotions going to get you out of pain? Read on.

Recall the information presented in Chapter 1 describing how our tendency to experience joy becomes sapped by chronic pain. Pain naturally grabs our attention because it's a warning signal of potential tissue damage. The brain can pay attention to only a limited number of things at once. Its attentional resources are finite, and staying alive (via paying attention to pain) is priority number one. Think of your attention capacity like slices of a pie: if, say, 8 of 12 slices are devoted to noticing pain sensations and their potential negative consequences (like not being as productive at work), not much is left for seeking out and enjoying joyful and meaningful activities. The more you back away from pleasurable activities that help you feel safe, happy, and at ease, the more you confirm your brain's erroneous belief that you're in danger.

You might say, as I did when I first learned about the research on reward system dysfunction in chronic pain, yeah, duh. If I feel like I always have a knife in my back (or shoulder, face, abdomen, or over my whole body), of course I'm not going to enjoy that campfire, movie, or hike as much as somebody without pain. And that's true. But here's the interesting thing: research suggests that paying attention to and enjoying pleasant sensations is a pathway to lowering your pain. Why? We've talked about the release of naturally occurring painkillers with positive feelings and about how positive feelings build resilience by helping you think and act in healthier ways. Another reason has to do with how the brain makes decisions. The brain has been called "predictive," meaning that it is always making guesses about what might happen next in a very complex world. Based on its guesses, it tries to help you make the best decisions you can, moment by moment, to keep you alive and well.

Your brain is very concerned with two survival strategies: (1) avoid dangers with fight-flight-freeze behaviors and (2) go after rewards. Let's unpack that a bit more. Sometimes you really do need to avoid dangers (a hot stove, a car speeding through a crosswalk, or, in our human ancestors' case, an attacking tiger or wolf). You also need to do a whole lot of other things *that feel good* to survive in this world: eat nutritious foods, do things to make sure you stay included in social groups (be kind and empathic, for example), and be creative and learn things (like languages or math). You need to both *avoid* dangers and *approach* rewards. Pain is really good at getting you to *fixate on avoiding dangers*. Actually too good. But *the brain can suppress pain* when an important reward is available, because doing so will help you *succeed* in getting the reward. If your aching shoulder felt a bit better, you'd be more likely to have a lively conversation with your spouse, that is, you would be more successful in getting a social reward (a deeper bond).

Let's explore this concept with another metaphor. Indulge me and picture a menu at a nice restaurant with "SURVIVAL" written at the top. Below that are various menu items that can help you live another day, including "avoid-danger" and "approach-reward" options. You're extremely curious to review them all and make the best choice. Much to your chagrin, pain is shining a flashlight on the avoid-danger options on the menu, making it hard to see the rewards. As a diner at a nice restaurant, you might get upset and say, *Wait! I want to see those other tasty options!* Pain replies, *Get those rewards later. Right now it's more important to run for your life. Look only at the one or two options I'm showing you.* Picture your brain looking at the menu too. It's trying to help you make a good decision about what to order. "Avoid danger" and "enjoy rewards" are competing for your brain's attention: *Pick me, pick me!* they cry. And your brain senses how certain you are that you would like the other delicious options, if only you could see them. With rewards in mind, your brain decides that pain is being a control freak and should have less influence on the situation. It decides that *pain should go down* so that the rewards can be illuminated too.

In other words, to pursue and consume a reward, it's most productive (you're most likely to have success in acquiring the reward) if your pain goes down. Indeed, scientists consistently observe that enjoying rewards lowers pain. For example, when researchers bring people into the laboratory and apply noxious (potentially dangerous) heat to their skin, when they're given a reward (like money) at the same time, their pain goes down. Out in the real world, when people with chronic pain experience positive events or feelings in their daily lives, they report lower pain. In a study I contributed to as a postdoctoral fellow at Johns Hopkins, when patients with rheumatoid arthritis practiced a savoring meditation designed to increase positive emotions (which you'll learn about in Chapter 7), they reported lower pain and showed more brain activity in areas of the reward system than those patients with rheumatoid arthritis who practiced a breathing meditation that didn't promote positive feelings.

Sadly, chronic pain can make the world so incredibly small. Social activities are exhausting, nothing feels fun anymore, it's hard to think straight, and it's just so tiring to put on a happy face for pain-free people who just don't get it. I understand. I've been there. Hear me out: Joy and meaning are important pathways out of chronic pain. They help teach the brain that you're safe and well. In this chapter, you'll identify sources of joy and meaning in your life and consider how you might use those resources more deeply and purposefully to benefit your pain symptoms. You'll hear about science-backed sources of joy, calm, and ease that can be sidelined by chronic pain so you can brainstorm new ways of experiencing pleasure. In so doing you'll rehabilitate your brain's reward system and help convince it that you're safe.

Strengths and Resilience

Let's start with your strengths and the positive influences that remain in your life despite pain. Looking back, a few lifelines that I held onto through my worst pain symptoms were lap swimming, yoga, dates with friends (as much as their concerned "How are you?" question would feel so darkly meaningless and I would robotically respond "Not too bad"), and the hopeful expectation that I would one day become pain-free. I was persistent in seeking pain relief, I got into psychotherapy, and I stayed in graduate school.

Although all may feel lost, I promise you it's not. You already have some tools. We all have sources of strength, resilience, and joy already present in our lives that we often discount or overlook, and you can build on them and consider new sources of reward.

REFLECT: How are you resilient? What are your greatest strengths? What are you most proud of? Who in your community is supporting you (friends, family, pets, physical therapists, doctors, spiritual or religious leaders)? What are you still doing that brings you joy and meaning despite the pain? Can you do more with your strengths? Write in a journal or in the blank lines below whatever comes to mind without censoring your- self. If writing isn't your thing, take a moment to close your eyes (if that's comfortable) and envision the answers to these questions. At the end of your reflections, appreciate the energy and effort you have devoted to taking care of your well-being in the areas you identify.

....

....

....

Science-Backed Sources of Pleasure and Happiness

Social Connection

As discussed in Chapter 2, a lack of social bonds is perceived by the ner- vous system as a threat. On the flip side, the presence of healthy social connection is a powerful source of reward and safety and thus provides pain relief. Scientific studies robustly confirm the intuitive notion that high-quality social connections (friendships, intimate relationships) pro- mote positive feelings. Further, we've learned that social belonging can relieve pain. For example, research has documented a significant rela- tionship between the number of friends people have and their ability to tolerate pain. Laughing with friends promotes the release of endogenous opioids (the body's natural painkillers) and increases pain threshold (the point at which we perceive pain in response to a potentially dangerous stimulus). Having a responsive, emotionally supportive partner has been shown to promote better pain outcomes in patients with chronic pain undergoing surgery (for instance, joint replacement). Research confirms that during painful procedures holding the hand of someone who cares about you lowers the pain perceived. Finally, when we spend time with people who engage in healthy behaviors (exercise, healthy diet, stress management) and encourage us to do the same, we're more likely to maintain healthy behaviors ourselves, which can promote health and longevity in the long term. Healthy social connection appears to relieve pain directly through the release of the body's natural painkillers, indirectly through enhanced reward system function (positive emotions), and via healthy behaviors.

REFLECT: I invite you to think about your positive social experiences. Bring to mind a time when you felt a sense of belonging, laughed with friends, felt loved by your spouse, or did a fun activity with friends. What were you thinking and feeling? What did you see, smell, touch, taste, and hear? What was your pain like? If comfortable, close your eyes and savor this memory. Register any benefits of this experience (improved well-being, reduced pain) in your body and mind now.

WHAT CAN I DO? Are you keeping up with social engagements despite the pain? Are you saying no to invitations to spend time with others because you fear the pain will ramp up? Do you feel safe and happy in your close (spousal) relationships? Can you think of ways you can improve your social well-being to benefit your pain?

Think of socializing as a pain-relief pill: you'll give your body an opportunity to release pain-reliving biochemicals and improve how well your reward system works in general. In Chapter 6 you'll find specific ways to build your social well-being.

Prosocial and Altruistic Behavior

Whenever we feel threatened (by chronic pain or other dangers), we naturally become self-focused. Our attention narrows to how to escape the problem. We easily become fixated on a self-focused narrative about how the pain emerged and what the (bleak) future may look like. Prosocial emotions (love, compassion, kindness) and behaviors (giving time, money, or support to others or social causes)—those that benefit others—are antidotes to this self-focused, fear-based frame. Indeed, Western science agrees with what wisdom and religious traditions across the globe have taught for quite a while: that giving to or doing things for others is more rewarding than doing things for oneself. Acting altruistically increases positive emotions and self-esteem and imbues our life with meaning, purpose, and value.

When my pain was at its very worst, I would experience glimmers of relief when I tried to focus on others rather than obsessing about myself. I thought if I can't get rid of the pain at least my life will have meaning. I'm reminded of a recent phone call I had with a dear friend during which I asked how her Mother's Day was. She replied that her four-year-old daughter was up at 3:00 a.m. because she was so excited to make breakfast in bed for Mom that she couldn't sleep! This adorable example shows how rewarding it is to give.

So what about prosocial behavior and pain? A series of recent studies showed that acting altruistically relieves pain. In one, cancer patients with chronic pain (volunteers) were randomly assigned to perform altruistic acts or self-focused acts over seven days. Fascinatingly, patients in the altruistic group showed a significantly greater reduction in pain. In a different experiment people who volunteered to do an altruistic activity experienced less laboratory-induced pain after doing it than those who declined to act altruistically, as well as those who were assigned it as a mandatory task. Another study showed that people who donated blood perceived significantly less pain during the blood draw than people who provided blood for their own benefit, despite the fact that the needle used for blood donation is far larger and thicker than the kind typically used at the doctor's office.

Research shows that we often look for happiness in all the wrong places. We think that buying material goods that we like will keep us happy. So, if it feels like focusing on generosity and other-focused activity isn't going to do much for your reward system, you're not alone. Yet studies suggest that other-focused generosity tends to promote happiness more than self-focused activity. For example, nationally representative survey data have shown that self-focused spending is unrelated to happiness while spending money on others (gifts and charity) is associated with greater happiness, even after accounting for total income. Related studies suggest that when employees receive a financial bonus at work, the extent to which they spend the money on others is more important to their happiness than the size of the bonus itself. Lastly, people randomly assigned to spend a financial windfall on others have been shown to experience a significantly greater boost in happiness than those assigned to spend it on themselves. The finding that altruism promotes happiness has been replicated in numerous labs around the world.

Research also robustly shows that what we put out into the world we get back. In other words, when we act to benefit others, we often get the same in return. Acting with compassion and kindness feels good in the moment (the "helper's high" or "warm glow" we get from giving) but also helps you build enduring social relationships that can support successfully navigating life with chronic pain. Part Three will help you build on your inherent prosocial traits and aspirations.

REFLECT: Recall a time that you showed kindness, understanding, forgiveness, compassion, or appreciation to another. Maybe you've offered tangible gifts in the past (a monetary gift or service). Maybe you tend to pause and express genuine appreciation for others' generosity and service (salespeople, caregivers, friends). Maybe you're kind in ongoing ways to your children, spouse, friends, or coworkers. Maybe you're devoted to taking care of your pets or the earth (a garden). Recall a prosocial memory with the five senses now. Recall any positive feelings that may have arisen, like warmth, ease, or happiness. Perhaps you were in touch with your own basic goodness and natural caring of others. Allow any positive feelings to fill your body now. Appreciate the goodness you extended to others now in this moment.

WHAT CAN I DO? Are there ways to increase other-focused kindness, care, and generosity in your life, for your own and others' benefit? His Holiness the 14th Dalai Lama calls this "enlightened self-interest": when we think and act prosocially, we ourselves benefit right along with those we help. For you, could prosocial feelings and activities be a pathway to experiencing reward and pain relief?

Spirituality and Self-Transcendence

Spiritual and/or religious practices can be deeply rewarding and meaningful. Spirituality is a broad concept (sometimes considered synonymous with religiosity) that involves a sense of connection to something larger than oneself (often termed *self-transcendence*). It could include a sense of the sacred and experiences of oneness with all things or a higher power (such as the universe, God, the earth). Self-transcendence is an important, if not fundamental, part of spiritual life. Psychologist and meditation teacher Tara Brach likens self-transcendence to the recognition of the self as a wave in the ocean: although each wave (person, being, creature) has its unique characteristics, it is a manifestation of and is not separate from the vast sea. When we experience ourselves as a manifestation of something boundless (God, the universe, nature) and feel that we inherently belong, we can experience an abiding sense of calm, ease, and joy. Indigenous wisdom traditions have long known our inherent belonging to the sacred and natural world.

Scientists are actively studying how to promote self-transcendent experiences in which we no longer feel small, separate, and vulnerable and instead feel inexorably connected with a larger whole and how those experiences impact our emotions and health, including pain. Meditation, nature contact, and psychedelics can elicit self-transcendent states, which are reviewed in Parts Three and Five. Self-transcendent emotions including awe (the feeling of being in the presence of something vast and mysterious), gratitude (consciously perceiving and appreciating the many benefits in our lives), and elevation (profound appreciation for the good works of others, like their virtue or artistic contributions) are other experiences that can take us beyond the self.

If you think about it, if fear is a driver of pain (because we feel vulnerable and need to protect ourselves), trusting our inherent belonging through a sense of oneness and nonseparation is a potent fear antidote and source of serenity, calm, and ease. I've worked with several clients for whom self-transcendence really matters. I've been told that gratitude meditation can provide pain relief in the moment. Being in nature or serving others can quiet the self-focused narratives about pain, danger, and upset. One found purpose in embodying her deepest, other-focused values of generosity and altruism, despite the suffering she had endured throughout her life. In my case I often reflect on how the separate, vulnerable self is an illusion: we do not exist apart from the air we breathe, the food we eat, or the trillions of microorganisms that live inside us and on our skin that we can't survive without.

REFLECT: Take a moment to reflect on your spirituality. Your spiritual life could be linked with a place of worship or religious community, or you might experience spirituality through nature, art, or other forms of beauty. Maybe you experience awe and mystery through reflecting on how minuscule the earth is in a vast universe. How are you spiritual or religious? What brings up a sense of awe for you? Do you touch into something sacred? If so, how?

EXERCISE

After considering these general questions, I invite you to recall a positive spiritual or religious memory, perhaps a time when you felt connected to a deity, a higher power, the universe, or the natural world; a time when you felt connected with something sacred, loving, or awe-inspiring. Recall this experience with the five senses, allowing any positive feelings such as peace, joy, ease, serenity, or trust to fill your body and mind now. Note any changes in your pain, either from the past or in this moment as you engage in this reflection. If you like, write them in the lines below or in a journal.

....

....

....

WHAT CAN I DO? Think about which spiritual or religious practices that are important to you, if any, have fallen off due to pain. Do spiritual or religious activities increase positive emotions, reduce your pain, or help you cope with it? Are you seeking a spiritual or religious life?

Sports and Other Physical Activity

Research shows that physical activity can increase positive emotions, reduce negative emotions, reduce inflammation, and improve self-confidence and social support (particularly in the case of interactive forms of exercise like team sports or group exercise). Physical activity and positive emotions can interact in an upward spiral: movement promotes positive emotions, and feelings of enjoyment emerging from the activity motivate us to keep doing it, in turn keeping positive emotions flow-ing. Unfortunately, exercise in our culture has often been constructed as a boring, nose-to-the-grindstone obligatory activity (like jogging on a treadmill in a packed gym). But our bodies have evolved to be in motion, and I think it's important to reframe physical activity as nourishing and fun. What do you like to do that involves physical activity? Garden-ing, walking, pickleball, dancing, yoga, soccer, hiking? Don't forget that doing a few body weight exercises at regular intervals throughout the day counts, as do activities of daily living like cleaning and yardwork.

Although you might fear that movement will make you feel worse, research indicates that exercise programs are safe for people with chronic pain and improve pain and function. People with chronic pain often ben-efit from working with a physical therapist who can help them pace their activity based on their own interest and situation. Pacing yourself means avoiding the extremes of over- and underexertion, including being inten-tional about building in rest breaks around your activity, slowly build-ing up your activity capacity over time, and saving up energy for things that you value most (like spending time with your kids or friends) when needed. A physical therapist or physical rehabilitation specialist can help you determine how to pace your activity so that you're on the right path. There will be more about physical activity in Part Four.

REFLECT: Think of a time when you were physically active in a way that felt fun or at least neutral. Maybe you were playing a sport, dancing, gardening, or taking a brisk walk outdoors. What did you feel, see, smell, and touch? Register any positive feelings or sensations associated with this experience in your mind and body now. Remember any reductions in pain that may have happened. Maybe the physical activity didn't feel particularly positive, but perhaps it felt neutral, doable, safe. Maybe you experienced a sense of accomplishment at the end. In your mind's eye, picture the experience and appreciate the effort you made and any ben-efits that resulted.

WHAT CAN I DO? Can you identify physical activities, however small, that are or could be nourishing to you? Is there a way to gradually increase your physical activity? What could you do today, tomorrow?

Music, Art, and Creativity

Listening to or making music, looking at or making art, and singing activate the brain's reward network and promote a release of the brain's natural painkillers. Many studies have documented the pain-relieving effects of music and the arts. For instance, vocal music therapy done regularly over several weeks (toning and humming, singing in a group, deep breathing, and vocal improvisation) has been shown to improve pain and stress management, mood, sense of belonging, self-confidence, and self-appreciation. Listening to pleasant music (versus neutral sounds) in a lab has been shown to lower pain and improve mobility task performance. Jane would do a "music meditation" to help herself get through pain and fatigue flares. She would lie in bed, close her eyes, and put on her favorite playlist. She would try to fully rest her attention on the sounds, moment by moment. She told me that this practice really comforted her in tough moments. Expressing yourself creatively through the arts, writing, cooking, gardening, games, carpentry, or anything else that allows for creative expression can activate positive emotions and a sense of meaning.

REFLECT: Think of a time when you experienced and appreciated beauty. Beauty could take any number of forms: art, music, theater, nature, literature, good comedy, film, something spiritual or religious, or even something scientific or mathematical that impressed and created a sense of awe in you. Perhaps when you listen to and/or sing a favorite song, a certain set of positive feelings (calm, nostalgia, playfulness) arises. Think of something personally meaningful to you now and contact that memory with the five senses. What happened physically, emotionally? Receive any positive feelings that arise in response to this reflection.

WHAT CAN I DO? Are there creative or artistic activities that you have or could try to activate positive emotions? Maybe you have some prior experience with creative expression that you'd like to revisit, or maybe it's the right time to challenge yourself to try something completely new. If you can do something creative in a group and/or with a teacher you like (singing in a choir, a pottery class), you'll get the combined rewards of social interaction and creative expression.

Contact with Nature

Humans evolved to interact with the natural world, yet we're increasingly spending most of our time indoors. Our bodies simply function better if we get out into nature. For instance, the ancient Japanese practice of forest bathing (mindfully savoring walks in the forest) has been shown in multiple studies to improve immune system functioning. Interacting with nature increases positive emotions, and as discussed previously, can inspire self-transcendent and spiritual experiences such as awe. Studies suggest that nature experiences reduce stress (recall how stress increases the sensitivity of the pain alarm) as well as mental fatigue. Spend more time outside, and I promise that you'll feel better.

REFLECT: Recall a compelling experience of contact with the natural world. It could be from childhood or something more recent. See if you can think of a time when you felt connected with the land, earth, or sea. Bring to mind the physical sensations that were happening, perhaps a breeze or mist on your face, solid ground beneath your feet, any sounds of waves or wind, wildlife. Notice any pleasant feelings that arise in your body as you bring this memory to mind. Notice any positive effects on your pain level from the past or during this exercise.

WHAT CAN I DO? Take a moment to reflect on how much "vitamin N" (that is, time in nature) you're getting. What activities draw you to the outdoors? How can you increase your connection with the natural world that holds and sustains us all? Are there things that you do indoors (exercise, resting) that you could do outside? You'll learn how to mindfully savor pleasant experiences, including nature experiences, in Part Three.

Hope and Positive Expectations

As discussed in the Introduction, expectations matter. Positive, hopeful expectations promote pain relief. Tragically, I've heard patients tell me that physicians, even those with little understanding of their situation, tell them they'd likely be in pain for the rest of their life and should just learn to accept it. It's truly maddening. Naturally such statements perpetuate negative expectations and reduce the motivation to lower pain via mental and behavioral strategies and to persist with a holistic pain care plan. The worsening of symptoms through negative expectations (and other negative experiences like a poor doctor–patient relationship) is known in the scientific literature as *nocebo*, which is the opposite of *placebo*.

REFLECT: What reasons do you have to be hopeful? What positive expectations do you have for your healing journey? What faith do you have that you will get better? Can you see yourself getting back to activities that you've given up because of your pain?

WHAT CAN I DO? If you have expectations that you'll only stay the same or get worse, can you pause and notice those expectations and view them as real (they're happening) but not the truth?

EXERCISE

As we conclude this chapter, take a few moments to reflect on what you've given up because of chronic pain.

What Have I Given Up?

Write what comes to mind, in the blank lines below or in a journal, describing whatever thoughts, feelings, or reactions come up without censoring yourself.

■ What sources of joy or meaning do you want to engage with but find challenging?

▪ How could you, even in the smallest way, start intentionally building more positive activities into your day?

....

....

....

▪ What in this chapter resonated most with you or felt important?

....

....

....

As you did for threats in Chapter 2, it may help to use a checklist to get a broad look at the science-backed sources of happiness that you think you could nurture as part of a holistic pain self-management plan. I'm guessing there is already a glimmer of each of these in your life.

My Resilience Factors

❏ Social connections: family, friends, and intimate relationships

❏ Benefiting others: kindness, compassion, and altruism

❏ Spirituality and self-transcendence

❏ Sports and physical activities

❏ Contact with nature

❏ Music, art, and creativity

❏ Hope and positive expectations

❏ Other

PART TWO

REDUCING THREATS AND FINDING SAFETY

Let's dive right into science-backed ways of getting your nervous system out of high alert and into a place of calm and safety. This part will introduce you to strategies that you can start using right away. Know that because your brain has essentially been "practicing" pain production, and gotten very good at it, it's going to take some repetition and time to retrain it. Be patient and persistent and trust that your efforts will improve your pain and well-being, even if the effects aren't apparent right away.

4

Working with Pain Sensations and Thoughts

Mindfulness-Based and Cognitive Approaches

Mindfulness practices are drawn from Buddhist psychology and broadly refer to the practice of paying attention in a nonjudgmental, open, and accepting way to whatever arises in your field of awareness, including pain sensations. Whatever presents itself in your consciousness, be it pain, pleasure, or something neutral, when you practice mindfulness you welcome it with kindness, acceptance, and love. Imagine a tiny baby, small child, or other precious and vulnerable being like a kitten or puppy. When it cries out, you hold it close and offer comfort and acceptance; you remain present and available to it and hear its cries with compassion. You don't cast it aside angrily, criticize, or blame it for struggling. This is the kind of attitude that mindfulness-based practices for pain encourage, and research shows that practicing mindfulness both formally (through sitting, standing, or walking meditation) and informally (by practicing mindful awareness in activities of daily life such as washing dishes or driving) can lower pain and improve quality of life. Volumes have been written on the use of mindfulness practices for chronic pain and illness (Jon Kabat-Zinn's *Full Catastrophe Living* is a good one).

Mindfulness for Pain

Why does mindfulness work? There are multiple mechanisms, but a key one is that it helps take the nervous system out of danger-alert mode by changing your relationship to physical sensations and thoughts. Your mind can contribute to nervous system hypersensitivity through all the fear-based, angry, and hopeless thoughts that arise in response to raw pain sensations. You feel the aversive sensation of pain, and the mind churns out thoughts: *What's wrong? This is my fault. Why did I spend all those years slumped over my desk? I probably can't work tomorrow. I might be in pain forever. There's no hope. I hate this. I'm a burden.* The brain takes these thoughts into account as it decides whether to keep producing pain. These kinds of thoughts are scary, thus increasing the likelihood that the brain will decide that it's best for your survival to keep you focused on potential dangers (via producing pain) rather than on resting and restoring (via stopping pain). Researchers sometimes call this process an "emotional enhancement of pain": proliferating thoughts help keep the nervous system stuck on making pain.

Note that it's only natural for the mind to produce unhelpful and fear-based thoughts, particularly in response to pain. Just as the body secretes enzymes, the mind secretes thoughts. If your mind is busy with imagined catastrophes, you're in good company. But you can get a handle on them. Ari sought therapy to deal with a new and shocking diagnosis of a chronic inflammatory condition. It brought on agonizing, periodic pain flares. He would get stuck rehashing the past, and his mind would spin stories about who was to blame. *Why did this happen? It's all my fault. I shouldn't have had so much to drink in college or let my stress get so out of control when I was clerking at that law firm. How could I have been so careless?! Maybe others are to blame. My coworkers are so toxic. If they hadn't created such a stressful environment at the office, maybe I wouldn't be here.* Over time he came to realize that these narratives were only compounding the pain. These thoughts were cutting him off from happiness, and so were the behaviors he fell into to try to take control, like searching for answers online. To get unstuck, he started labeling his familiar thought trains with television channels. Lightheartedly he would note, *oh, looks like I'm watching channel 5! Who turned that on?!* This approach helped him see the story for what it was: a bunch of thought forms that were neither factual nor helpful. It might help you to use a mental image as Ari did to get unstuck from your mental stories, like movie plots appearing on a blank screen. The mind is constantly generating thoughts and stories, but you don't need to get lost in them. Watch how they arise and pass.

As Ari's experience shows, the goal of mindfulness is not to make thoughts disappear. The key is to relate to thoughts differently. Another commonly used analogy is to imagine your thoughts as leaves on a stream. You're sitting on a riverbank and watching them float by. Similarly, your mind is like a clear-blue sky with various weather patterns (storms, cute and fluffy clouds) moving through. Some weather patterns (thought forms) are deeply compelling and captivating, whereas others are relatively mild and uninteresting. As you adopt this mindful attitude toward physical sensations (pain), thoughts, and feelings that arise, you can lower your body's overall threat level. Mindfulness can be challenging since it's exactly the opposite of what you may feel like doing; we're wired to turn away from what's difficult. But turning toward difficulty, and in so doing letting your nervous system know that you're OK, you'll tip your physiology and emotional well-being in the direction of safety.

EXERCISE

Let's pause for a mindfulness practice. I invite you to read the steps one by one. After reading each instruction close your eyes, if comfortable, and do the practice for up to a few minutes.

1. Set an intention: I take a moment now to pause and care for my well-being. Rather than going to war with my experience, I intend to practice peace.

2. Ground yourself: Notice sensations and points of contact between your body and chair or floor, wherever you're seated, standing, or lying down. Feel the earth supporting you now. Imagine yourself as an old, wise, strong tree, with roots extending downward, deep into the ground. Contact a sense of groundedness, connection, and stability.

3. Concentrate mindfully: Rest your attention on an anchor of your choice:

the sensations of breath moving in and out of your belly, the arising and passing of sounds, perhaps an area of your body (hands or feet) that is pain free. Rest your attention on this anchor and as thoughts, feelings, and physical sensations arise, gently notice and label them (thinking, planning, worrying) and bring your attention back to your anchor. See if you can keep a nonjudgmental, loving attitude toward yourself and whatever shows itself. Spend a couple of minutes engaging in this concentration practice.

4. Appreciate yourself: Thank yourself for the effort you've put forth to practice mindful presence and trust that you've sent signals of peace and safety to your nervous system.

Through this practice it becomes easier to see that our thoughts create, in the words of meditation teacher and psychotherapist Dr. Tara Brach, a virtual reality. We can notice the virtual world and gently come out of it by returning to the anchor. Please note that if when you practice mindfulness you feel flooded (highly overwhelmed) by scary and even traumatic thoughts or feelings, it's not a good time to practice mindfulness meditation by yourself. Rather, seek the support of a therapist, meditation teacher, or meditation group for support.

EXERCISE

A practice that you can do in addition to mindfulness is to explicitly challenge habitual, unhelpful thoughts by writing them down and then replacing them with alternative, more accurate and helpful thoughts. Whenever I'm caught in a sea of thoughts, I try to joke to myself about how ridiculous they would sound if I had to yell them out through a loudspeaker for all to hear. That's kind of what this exercise is getting at. I invite you to identify your habitual thoughts below and come up with alternative thoughts that may be more helpful and accurate. The examples that follow reflect what I often hear from therapy clients and that I've experienced myself:

....

....

....

....

Habitual thought: *It's hopeless. I'll never get better.*

More accurate thoughts: *I'm on a journey toward healing, and I know that healing and well-being are within my reach. People around the world are healing from chronic pain every day. Each chronic pain situation is unique, and I'm figuring out my specific recipe for healing. I'm proud of the steps I've taken today to live meaningfully and remain an active participant in my life despite pain. I'm going to stay persistent.*

Habitual thought: *I'm a burden. I'm letting other people down. Ultimately they'll stop loving me.*

More accurate thoughts: *I am worthy of the love and care that others give me. It's OK to need and ask for help. It doesn't mean I'm weak or defective. I don't buy into ableist messages that invisible illnesses are unacceptable. At some point in their lives, every human will become ill and need the care and support of others. I give to others as well, and I don't discount that; for example, I give love, care, empathy, and encouragement to others. When others express love and care toward me, I believe them, and I allow myself to trust their love.*

Habitual thought: *I've gone into a pain and fatigue flare. What if this is my new normal?!*

More accurate thoughts: *This is temporary. I'm in a flare, which totally sucks, but I will come out of it. I'm going to focus on my self-care plan, refrain from googling health information, and trust that I'll be OK.*

I invite you to identify and challenge habitual thoughts below:

Habitual thought: ....

More accurate thoughts: ....

Habitual thought: ....

More accurate thoughts: ....

Habitual thought: ....

More accurate thoughts: ....

FOR MORE INFORMATION ON MINDFUL PRACTICE

Mindfulness-based interventions have proliferated, and there are so many resources available for regular practice. Your best shot at retraining your brain is through practicing regularly, and guided audio recordings or organized classes are a huge help. Here are some of my favorite resources:

- Smartphone Applications: Calm, Insight Timer (follow teachers Ruth King, Jack Kornfield, Joseph Goldstein, and Tara Brach), Headspace (don't forget *Curable*, which I mentioned previously—many mindfulness-based exercises are embedded in it)
- The Insight Meditation Community of Washington: *www.imcw.org* (talks, meditations, and articles)
- Mindfulness-Based Stress Reduction through Palouse Mindfulness (a free course): *https://palousemindfulness.com*
- Sounds True: *www.soundstrue.com*
- University of California San Diego Center for Mindfulness: *https://cih.ucsd.edu/mindfulness*
- If you have a rheumatic disease like arthritis, check out the Johns Hopkins mindfulness in rheumatology program that my colleagues Dr. Dana DiRenzo (a rheumatologist at the University of Pennsylvania) and Dr. Neda Gould (director of the mindfulness program at Johns Hopkins) and I developed: *https://mindfulness.hopkinsrheumatology.org*
- Banyan: An online meditation community that you can access from anywhere, with excellent teachers at an affordable price: *https://banyantogether.com*

Challenging Internalized Chronic Pain Stigma

Use the techniques in this section to challenge self-defeating beliefs that may have cropped up because of chronic pain stigma. Consider Elyse, who was receiving accommodations at her workplace to help her deal with fibromyalgia. Her company allowed her to reduce her work hours on weeks that she wasn't feeling well. But she hesitated to use her accommodations for fear of being seen as weak or being accused by colleagues of "faking it." Even worse, when she did use her accommodations, she *felt* weak. She would question herself: *Are my symptoms really that bad? Is it*

all in my head? I can't seem to just power through. What's wrong with me?!
We worked together to help her see these thoughts in a more accurate
light: not as truths, but as products of harmful, inaccurate societal messages about people living with invisible disabilities. She replaced these
inaccurate thoughts with accurate ones: *I'm not weak; I'm living with a*
health condition. I'm the expert on what I'm experiencing, and it's my right
to trust my own judgment. Only I know how I feel and what I need. I'll be
better and more able to help others if I use all the tools that I know help me.
Releasing the shame associated with the "I'm weak" narrative, Elyse felt
more empowered to enact her pain self-management plan. She suffered
less and noticed that her new beliefs shifted her emotions away from the
negative (shame, anger at self) and toward the positive (self-acceptance
and kindness). This was a fundamental step in Elyse's "upward spiral"
toward pain recovery.

Social conditioning is intensely powerful: if you find yourself accus-
ing yourself of being weak, unmotivated, fabricating, lazy, incapable,
unproductive, or even entitled, you've bought into harmful stereotypes
about people living with chronic pain. See these thoughts for what they
are (harmful stereotypes that you've inadvertently absorbed) and replace
them.

Pain Reprocessing Therapy:
An Exciting New Treatment

Pain reprocessing therapy, or PRT, is an exciting new science-backed
treatment for chronic pain, which works by helping people change their
beliefs about the causes of chronic pain. It elegantly brings together pain
neuroscience education (which you learned about in Part One), mindfulness (which we just reviewed), and a technique called *safety reappraisal*,
which refers to relabeling pain sensations as safe (that is, reflective of a
misfiring of the alarm system rather than a problem in the body). Safety
reappraisal in PRT borrows from safety reappraisal in the treatment of
panic attacks, where people learn to label physical sensations arising
during a panic attack that feel dangerous (sweaty palms, racing heart,
palpitations) as harmless. One of the developers of PRT, Alan Gordon,
a licensed clinical social worker, was a former intractable pain sufferer

himself who dove into the neuroscience of pain in an effort to cure his own widespread pain condition. You can read all about Gordon's journey and PRT in his excellent book *The Way Out: A Revolutionary, Scientifically Proven Approach to Healing Chronic Pain.*

Critically, PRT begins with helping people debunk their inaccurate beliefs that their chronic pain must be caused by a problem in the body (like a slipped disc) and understand that a hypersensitive alarm system could be the cause. PRT therapists help patients look at their own unique situation by reviewing prior scans, previous diagnoses, and learned associations and beliefs (for example, "My back hurts when I stand therefore there must be a structural problem in my back") and help them identify evidence that their pain could in fact be caused by nervous system hypersensitivity. This helps people buy into the notion that their pain can be lowered or eliminated by retraining the danger (pain) alarm to fire less frequently. Participants then begin a therapist-guided practice known as *somatic tracking,* which involves (1) mindfully noticing painful sensations with a lighthearted, curious mindset and (2) labeling those sensations as safe through self-talk ("This is safe, this is OK, there's nothing wrong in my body"). You can try a somatic tracking practice yourself at the Pain Psychology Center's website (see the box below). The developers argue that with time, as people shift their perspective on pain sensations from danger signals to unpleasant sensations that are in fact safe, chronic pain will subside.

PAIN REPROCESSING THERAPY RESOURCES

- Learn more, take an online workshop, or find a PRT-trained therapist at *www.painreprocessingtherapy.com.*
- Recommended Reading: *The Way Out: A Revolutionary, Scientifically Proven Approach to Healing Chronic Pain* by Alan Gordon.
- Practice somatic tracking and other skills using the Pain Psychology Center's website, *www.painpsychologycenter.com/how-it-works.*
- The smartphone app *Curable* is aligned with the principles of PRT.
- *In Health: A New Approach to Chronic Pain Recovery* is an online program based on PRT and modern pain neuroscience that is covered by several major insurance plans (*www.lin.health*).

What does the science say about PRT? To the best of my knowledge just one trial has been completed, which was published in 2022 in the journal *JAMA Psychiatry* and presents almost astounding results. At the end of the trial, two-thirds of participants in the PRT condition (66%), all with chronic back pain, reported elimination or near elimination of that pain, with improvements mostly maintained over one-year follow-up. In the placebo control group, just 20 percent of participants reported elimination or near elimination of pain (speaking to the power of positive expectations and other placebo factors in pain treatment, like having contact with a therapist), and just 10 percent in treatment as usual (no extra intervention except completing study measures, like questionnaires). The mechanism underlying improvement was a change in the belief that pain reflects tissue damage. PRT also produced favorable changes in brain functioning. Importantly, this trial focused on people with chronic back pain believed to be nociplastic (pain completely caused by nervous system hyperexcitability). Future research has yet to determine how effective PRT is for other pain conditions beyond chronic back pain, such as pain occurring with inflammatory bowel disorders, endometriosis, and sickle cell anemia. Nervous system hyperexcitability is present in a wide variety of chronic pain conditions though, and I think this treatment holds a great deal of promise for many people with pain. For the record I have no affiliation with the PRT developers. I just genuinely think it's a neat treatment grounded in the modern neuroscience of pain.

To sum up the key points from this chapter, our thoughts and beliefs about pain can be a source of threatening information that can ramp up the danger alarm. You can reduce your overall threat level by reducing emotional reactivity to pain through mindfulness, challenging fear-based thoughts, and offering yourself messages of encouragement and safety instead and by recognizing that chronic pain sensations are in fact safe (they're your brain misfiring, not accurate messages telling you about real tissue damage). Check out the online resources in the box on page 64 for additional support with safety reappraisal of pain sensations. As always, consult with your care team as you think about using new pain treatments such as PRT.

5

Addressing Trauma

As mentioned in Chapter 2, traumatic experiences often kick up the threat detection branch of the nervous system. Trauma history is far more prevalent in people who live with chronic pain than in people who don't, and the link between trauma and chronic pain is well established scientifically. When our sense of safety is violated by single traumas (natural disasters, medical traumas) or those ongoing (discrimination, emotional or physical abuse and neglect), the nervous system orchestrates itself as best it can to help us escape and prevent such threats from happening again. Our danger surveillance system, which includes pain and inflammation, can get kicked into high gear.

If you've experienced trauma (and very many people have), you aren't doomed to sickness. On the contrary. If you can identify trauma as something that has impacted you in important ways, you've taken a powerful step in figuring out your unique recipe for healing chronic pain. Trauma treatment could be an important part of your holistic pain treatment plan.

Let's talk more about what trauma can look like. Something can be obviously traumatic (a natural disaster or combat injury), or more subtle. Ongoing microaggressions and microinvalidations (slights like "You don't look sick" or "Where are you from?" or "You're so articulate!") on a day-to-day basis threaten our sense of safety and accumulate over time. Historical trauma (genocide, slavery) can impact the health and well-being of future generations. Ongoing racialized traumatic stress can have a weathering effect that manifests as physical, emotional, and psychological distress. Toxic relationship dynamics with other adults (intimate partners, family members, bosses) in which we feel criticized, invisible, devalued, or abandoned ramp up the alarm system. Even if we don't fully register that a relationship dynamic is hurtful to us, the body knows better, because it's just so good at figuring out that something isn't OK.

Let's zoom in on childhood, a long and vulnerable period in which the brain develops rapidly and we're wholly dependent on others for survival. Our brains continue developing in crucial ways into our early 20s in response to our experiences, a scenario that affords immense potential for our species (we can launch ourselves into outer space, for example), yet also renders us enormously vulnerable. The developing brain is highly plastic (malleable) and readily organizes itself in response to its environment, which might be safe and predictable, or it might be threatening and unpredictable. Whatever environment we're born into, the first and most central challenge we face in infancy and childhood is making sure we stay close to an adult who can nurture and protect us. Initially, of course, we have no idea how relationships (key sources of safety over our lifespan) are supposed to work. Through trial and error with our early caregivers (typically parents), we learn what behaviors get our needs for connection and protection met and which behaviors leave us rejected and alone. As a child, being alone is the ultimate threat (because we can't survive without an adult), so we'll do absolutely anything to keep the caregiver close. We develop a relationship template, or roadmap, based on our first experiences and then apply it in adult intimate relationships and even friendships.

Often the template we develop isn't so helpful or accurate when it comes to functioning well in adult relationships. Families are embedded in what can be dysfunctional intergenerational patterns and within society writ large, with its array of problems that can impact parents' ability to bond with and protect their children (colonialism, gun violence, racism and white supremacy, stigmatization of mental health care, land theft, police brutality, the climate crisis, and a general lack of economic supports available for families, to name a few). For whatever collection of reasons, your caregivers might not have known how to affirm, protect, and connect with you in general and during difficult moments.

If they were addicted to substances, abusive, neglectful, critical, judgmental, withdrawn, self-absorbed, emotionally dysregulated, (fill in the blank), you may have developed negative and inaccurate beliefs about yourself (I'm not lovable), felt responsible for the problems in your family, or thought your feelings didn't matter. Maybe you've carried these beliefs and associated behavioral patterns into your adult relationships, and you struggle to feel secure, at ease, and loved. Maybe you're tolerating harmful behavior (manipulation, abuse), or you might keep others at arm's length to try to stay safe (by isolating yourself or hiding your feelings). Or maybe you tend to act aggressively and put others down to try to feel secure. Whatever the collection of strategies, they're fed by the same root: fear.

Why does this matter for healing chronic pain? In scientific literature, attachment difficulties have been linked with disease processes, including pain severity. Sometimes attachment issues and their

RACIAL TRAUMA

Racial trauma is pervasive, and there is no cure-all without eliminating structural racism. Therapy with a culturally competent provider can yield a supportive space to process your experiences and build tools to cope with ongoing racialized stress, including ways of challenging internalized racism, defined as believing and acting as if the misinformation perpetuated by oppressive societal structures were true. As presented by Black experts, supportive approaches include:

- Consistently building racial pride (celebrate your race and culture all year long, such as through the arts, knowing your group's history, and ignoring White standards of success, intelligence, and beauty and instead forming standards within your own group)
- Joining safe spaces with other members of your race, such as communities that focus on a particular hobby or activity (gardening groups or book clubs)
- Limiting social media use, particularly content that documents violence toward members of your community
- Setting aside time each day for self-care (meditation, walks in nature, whatever feels nourishing to you)

subsequent "reenactment," to use a psychodynamic term, in adult relationships fly under the radar, and people don't notice how their alarm system is constantly ramped up, scanning for relational threats (criticism, rejection, lack of needed intimacy or support). Relationships should be an enduring source of joy and safety, and yet we're so often playing out our self-protective strategies that only drive us apart and feed our fears. Chapter 6 includes more about nurturing authentic, healthy relationships.

Treating Trauma

If the discussion in this chapter resonates with you, consider getting into therapy with a trauma specialist. Several online therapist directories are out there, including Inclusive Therapists, TherapyDen, Psychology Today, and Zencare, in which you can search for providers by your insurance, location, and provider specialty. You can also ask your primary care doctor for referrals. Trauma specialists often have training in one or more evidence-based trauma treatments, including:

- Eye movement desensitization and reprocessing (EMDR), a multistep treatment that involves exploring trauma memories while focusing on another point of focus at the same time, such as eye movements
- Cognitive processing therapy, with emphasis on identifying and changing unhelpful beliefs related to trauma
- Prolonged exposure, with emphasis on gradually approaching safe but feared memories, situations, and feelings that have been avoided
- Somatic experiencing, with emphasis on opening to physical sensations and related emotions in the body, gradually tolerating and accepting those sensations, and contacting inner sensations that feel safe and reassuring

Group therapy for trauma can also be very effective, as it provides the unique opportunity to connect and learn from others who have gone through similar experiences. Group therapy is usually more cost-effective than individual therapy. You can search for groups in the online directories mentioned earlier as well.

You might notice that part of you wants to start therapy whereas another part feels scared or hesitant. That's normal. It can feel scary to think about looking more deeply at previous or ongoing painful experiences. A skilled therapist will be able to foster a collaborative alliance with you; move at your pace; create a safe, culturally sensitive, and nonjudgmental space for exploration; and help you build inner resources using their specialized training. Getting into therapy does not mean you're weak. On the contrary. It reflects how strong you are: it's harder to turn toward emotional pain and to heal and work through it than it is to keep turning away from it. Doing your own emotional work will benefit your well-being along with the well-being of those around you.

In summary, as mentioned throughout this book, we each have a unique combination of factors that contribute to our pain. If prior or ongoing trauma is threatening your nervous system, treating the trauma though therapy might be a major part of your pathway out of chronic pain.

6

Cultivating Healthy Relationships and Belonging

Humans have long survived in groups and can't do life alone. So it's no surprise that the brain perceives a lack of interdependent, healthy, and supportive relationships as a threat. The term "interdependence" describes loving and respectful relationships in which each party can directly express their needs and feelings and have those expressions met with compassion and understanding. Each person gives and receives support, maintains a sense of autonomy and independence, and at the same time experiences a deep sense of belonging and what relationship experts Drs. John and Julie Gottman call "we-ness," a feeling of being part of a team. Relationships along these lines are an enduring source of positive emotions (including feelings of security and safety), which can alleviate pain.

I don't need to tell you that chronic pain imposes a profound challenge on close relationships. Here I discuss some relationship-enhancing principles that apply to people with and without chronic pain, as well as strategies that apply to chronic pain specifically.

Identify and Change Old Patterns

As noted in Chapter 5, in the past you may have developed certain ways of being in relationships that kept you safe (like pleasing, acting aggressively, or keeping your feelings to yourself). You can become aware of these patterns and replace them. After recognizing them you can honor the purpose they once served (protection), thank them for trying to help you, recognize that they no longer serve you, and practice new ways of nurturing safe and authentic closeness with others.

REFLECT: When you feel anxious, angry, down on yourself, or uncertain in an interpersonal situation, what's your go-to strategy? Take a moment to reflect on the following.

Do you

- fawn—please and placate other people while suppressing your own needs and wants;
- fight, acting angrily and aggressively through your speech or behavior, such as through blaming, boasting, or criticizing;
- flee—withdraw, disengage, isolate yourself, and/or dissociate through television, the internet, substances, or work; or
- pursue and attach, compulsively seeking attention and validation from others, in person or online through "likes"?

Next, explore the following.

- When I feel down, threatened, or insecure, what am I needing? What do I long for?

Ninety-nine times out of 100, we need love, security, to trust that we're enough exactly as we are, and to trust that we belong to others and to our world.

In the words of psychologist and meditation teacher Tara Brach, our protective strategies are like a space suit, a covering, and underneath it is our true and authentic self that longs to give and receive love. What does that mean? Being open and vulnerable in relationships, expressing our needs clearly, trusting our goodness and worth, being forgiving and compassionate toward others, and consistently engaging in the difficult task of having hard and honest conversations is our life's work.

Tap into Your Compassionate, Wise Self

When you notice a challenging feeling arise, pause and label it. Depending on what you notice, label it with feeling words like *fear, shame, anger,* or *sadness.* Take a deep breath and imagine caring for that feeling in the same way you would a small child or animal in distress. Rather than suppressing or fighting against the feeling, allow it. What message would the most loving person, pet, ancestor, or spiritual figure offer you in this moment? Then ask yourself: What do I need? What do I need to trust? What do I need to communicate?

This reflection will help you tap into your inner wisdom and guide your interactions with others from a place of compassion for all.

Set Healthy Boundaries

If you tend to suppress your feelings to please others, work on setting healthy boundaries. Stifling your own emotions and erasing yourself keeps your physiology in high-stress mode. Negative feelings of resentment, isolation, and sadness can easily build up inside. As one of my professors stated flatly during my first counseling class in graduate school, suppressed feelings leak out. They can leak out in the form of physical symptoms, depression and anxiety, passive aggression, and inauthenticity. On an extremely practical level, try using words like those shown below in conversations where you find yourself feeling pulled to placate others or struggling to express your needs:

- "I'm not sure what I think about that right now. I'll take some time to think about it and get back to you."
- "It's not OK with me to be spoken to that way. I need to be spoken to kindly and with respect."

- "Thanks for asking me. I'll be able to start working on this in two weeks, when my schedule is lighter."
- "When you're looking at your phone, I feel disconnected from you, and I really want to connect and spend time together after work because I care a lot about our relationship. Would you mind trying to be more present with me in the evenings?"
- "I need some time to take care of myself. Would you mind watching the kids two mornings a week for an hour so I can get out and walk?"
- "Thanks for sharing that with me, and that sounds really hard. This issue sounds like something that would best be dealt with through the support of a professional."
- "I'd love to help, but I'm not available."
- "When _____ happens, I notice that I feel _____. Would you mind doing _____?"

Nurture the Good

In the words of Vietnamese monastic and Buddhist teacher Thich Nhat Hanh, just as a flower needs sunlight and water to thrive, so, too, do loving relationships. If we don't intentionally nurture our shared love, it will die. One or more partners living with a chronic condition makes this even more crucial. Science confirms intuitive wisdom on how to water the seeds of love in relationships.

Frequently Express Appreciation

Saying "Thanks so much for taking out the trash!", showing affection and admiration ("I love you so much!" and "You're so accomplished; I'm so proud of you!") to important people in your life and toward those you'd like to become closer to goes a long way toward making connections. Put simply, we like and care for others who like and care about us. This is an example of the Dalai Lama's concept of enlightened self-interest. Express love, and everyone wins. When you can, try to make your feedback specific to something and beyond the general "Great job!" or "Love you!"

Challenge Yourself to Share Your Inner Life

Disclosure begets disclosure and deepens connection. So share feelings, hopes, perspectives, and past experiences with others. Avoid the extreme of overdisclosure, however, because that can promote disconnection. In conversations aim to disclose just a little bit more about yourself than what the other person has just disclosed to you.

Manage Conflict Wisely

When you notice yourself feeling angry, adopt a win-win mentality. Rather than adopting a me-versus-you mindset when things get heated, approach conflict with the question "What can I say and do that will maximize the likelihood that we'll work this out?" Pause and ask yourself if what you're about to say is true, kind, helpful, and likely to improve on silence.

Assume the Good

Dr. Becky Kennedy, a clinical psychologist, recommends that we take the "most generous interpretation" when considering another person's behavior. If someone in your life is acting in a hurtful or irresponsible way, see if you can make the most generous and compassionate interpretation before jumping to blame. Remember that people who cause suffering are suffering. Use this template: "I notice _____. What's going on for you? Help me understand."

Validate Feelings

Not all behaviors are OK, but all feelings are. When someone shares a feeling, even if it doesn't totally make sense to you, use phrases like

- "Thanks for sharing how you feel with me."
- "I can understand feeling that way."
- "I hear that you're feeling _____."
- "I care about how you're feeling, and thanks for telling me."
- "When I was in a similar situation, I also felt that way."

- Show compassion and solidarity with phrases like "That sounds really hard."
- "That's really rough, I get it."
- "I'm really sorry you're going through this, and I'm right here with you."

Help Others Understand
How They Can Help You with Chronic Pain

There is a roadmap for how significant others in your life (close friends, intimate partners, parents) can best help you manage your pain. The best way that they can respond to your pain and the emotional suffering associated with it is to

- show compassion;
- validate your feelings;
- support your efforts to engage in "well behaviors" such as exercise, socializing, and meditation;
- avoid inadvertently encouraging "sick behaviors" such as resting excessively, social media scrolling, relying only on pharmaceuticals for pain management as opposed to sticking to a holistic treatment plan; and
- work on their own reactions to the pain (sadness, fear) and their own mental well-being through their own therapy.

Here are some practical tips:

- Share your pain management goals with significant others and ask them to help encourage you, without making it their responsibility. For example, "I'm setting a new goal to get to the gym four times a week. I think some encouragement would really help me stick to the plan. Would you be willing to help encourage me and, if I'm not sticking to the plan, point it out?"
- Say "I don't need you to fix this for me. Right now I really need a hug and a shoulder to cry on. Your love and presence are all that I need right now. Thanks for being here."

- Say "I'm sure it's hard for you to see me in pain. How are you doing? What are you needing?"
- Say "I recently learned that when family members of people living with pain get into counseling, everyone benefits. I'm wondering if you might be interested in having a space to process everything that's going on related to my chronic pain and how it affects us. What do you think about that?"
- On days when your pain is lower than usual, use the opportunity to express love and care for others, in whatever way feels good to you (completing household tasks, doing something nice for your spouse).

Setting Boundaries around Chronic Pain Issues

As you know all too well, it's important to set healthy boundaries when it comes to your chronic pain condition specifically. Boundaries are needed to effectively manage your social life and to respond to others' comments about your condition, particularly when they're stigmatizing. Here are some examples:

- "I'd like to attend, and thanks for inviting me. I'm not able to make it, but I'd definitely like to try to hang out another time!"
- "I appreciate you suggesting that. I'm figuring out the next steps in my treatment plan with my treatment team."
- "Sure, I'll plan to go to that event with you a few months from now. I also want to share that my health can be unpredictable. If I need to cancel at the last minute, it's because I'm not feeling well unexpectedly, not because I don't want to be there. Thanks for your understanding! I'm really looking forward to seeing you."
- "My pain treatment plan involves avoiding alcohol and certain foods. Let's talk about something else!"
- "No one's pain is 'all in their head.' Please remember that all pain is real and stop questioning people's descriptions of their pain because it's harmful."
- "Even though you can't see it, my pain is real. People living with chronic pain often go through periods when they're very active

and don't look sick. I still need supports and accommodations to keep myself as well as possible."

- "If my pain flares up, sometimes I take longer than usual to respond to texts. If I'm delayed, it's not because I don't want to keep talking or don't value our friendship. Thanks for your understanding!"

Last but not least, if people start interviewing you about everything you've tried for your pain and ask if you've tried yoga, change the subject.

Join a Chronic Pain Support Group

Chronic pain support groups can help foster a sense of belonging and common humanity, that is, the experience of knowing you're not alone in your experience. They provide an opportunity to receive support and encouragement as well as give it to others, both of which can be pain-relieving. Having a supportive group of others who "get it" can help the body feel safer, and it can be a forum for a healthy exchange of ideas and strategies. Many groups can be found online. Find groups at the U.S. Pain Foundation's Pain Connection program (*https://painconnection. org/support-groups*) or the American Chronic Pain Association (*www. acpanow.com/support-groups.html*). You can also go to *Psychology Today*'s website (*www.psychologytoday.com*) and search for pain support groups.

Know What Unhealthy Relationships Look Like

Everything you've read in this chapter assumes you're in or cultivating healthy relationships that aren't abusive. Unhealthy relationship patterns can be hard to spot, and if you are in an unhealthy or abusive relationship, it's vital that you get help to protect both your physical and emotional well-being. Studies show that exposure to domestic or intimate partner abuse (including coercive, controlling, threatening, or violent behavior) significantly increases the risk of experiencing chronic pain. Here are some warning signs of an unhealthy relationship.

Your partner or other significant person in your life:

- insults, criticizes, belittles, or demeans you and may disguise these comments as jokes ("I was just kidding; can't you take a joke?");
- tries to isolate and keep you away from your loved ones;
- tries to control any aspect of your behavior, such as how you spend your time, and may retaliate (for example, by giving you the silent treatment) if you spend time away from them with friends or family;
- gets in the way of your taking care of your health, such as by discouraging you to attend doctor's appointments;
- trivializes your feelings;
- threatens you in any way;
- controls your access to money (such as through an "allowance");
- tells you that you're "too sensitive" or blames you for problems in the relationship, while refusing to take responsibility for their role;
- withholds affection and affirmation;
- accuses you of being self-centered and unsympathetic to their needs when you disagree or advocate for yourself;
- engages in any kind of physical abuse, sexual abuse or coercion, or digital abuse (harassing or embarrassing you online);
- threatens to hurt themselves or someone else if you leave them;
- breaks things, including possessions that you value; and
- is dishonest and defensive about an addiction for which they will not seek help.

You feel:

- like you're walking on eggshells for fear of your partner's anger or rage;
- afraid to speak up for yourself, advocate for yourself, or disagree with your partner;
- that you've given up things that you value;
- that your partner doesn't support your interests and goals outside of the relationship;
- ashamed or guilty;
- hopeless and powerless;
- unloved, unwanted, or abandoned;

- like you need to be more passive and placating than you would be with other people; and
- that you focus nearly all your energy on your partner.

It's never OK for someone to treat you with cruelty, ever. This list of behaviors isn't exhaustive. If you suspect that you may be in an unhealthy or abusive relationship, consult the National Domestic Violence Hotline's website (*www.thehotline.org*) and the One Love Foundation (*www.joinonelove.org*) for more information, examples of abusive behavior, and resources. For immediate support, call the National Domestic Violence Hotline at 800-799-7233, or text START to 88788.

FOR MORE INFORMATION ON HEALTHY RELATIONSHIPS

Deepening Intimate Relationships

The Gottman Institute: A Research-Based Approach to Relationships: *www.gottman.com*

Chronic Pain Support Groups

Pain Connection: *https://painconnection.org/support-groups*

American Chronic Pain Association: *www.acpanow.com/support-groups.html*

For caregivers: *https://uspainfoundation.org/uspfevents/caregivers-support-group*

Setting Healthy Boundaries

Nedra Tawwab's (*www.nedratawwab.com*) book *Set Boundaries, Find Peace*

Domestic and Intimate Partner Violence

National Domestic Violence Hotline at 800-799-7233, or text START to 88788.

The One Love Foundation on recognizing unhealthy relationships: *www.joinonelove.org/signs-unhealthy-relationship*

PART THREE

FINDING JOY AND LIVING MEANINGFULLY

Now that you've learned about various ways to help move your alarm system out of high-alert mode by calming and addressing different kinds of threats, you can discover ways of enhancing your brain's reward system. The reward system helps you feel positive emotions and be motivated to do things that are meaningful and important to you. It releases pain-relieving biochemicals. Research shows that with intentional practice we can improve how well the reward system works.

We're going to explore several approaches that are backed by wisdom traditions (for instance, Buddhism) and Western science. Rest assured that these methods of resourcing positive emotions have nothing to do with the notion that if we "just think positively" or mask negative experiences with pleasures we'll be OK (what has been called "toxic positivity").

You may notice an immediate increase in well-being or a reduction in pain when you try these strategies. More likely, however, it will take many repetitions. The brain has been "practicing" pain for so long that it may take a bit of time to quiet the pain signal via positive emotions. Be patient with yourself and trust that your efforts, sustained over time, will pay off.

7

Savoring

When something good happens, do you pause and savor it? Do you allow your body and mind to luxuriate in the positive? Or do you give it a quick nod and tumble forward onto the next thing? If you're like most people in our speedy society, it's the latter. The dominant culture conditions us to race and produce and control things in our lives rather than let go and be open to receive the good, enjoy what we have, slow down, and feel alive. Biologically, even without chronic pain in the equation, our brains are biased toward the negative because our ancestors who fixated on threats (tigers lurking in the woods) were more likely to survive and reproduce than those who didn't. You might go an entire year at work with only glowing reviews from supervisors, but that one piece of negative and constructive feedback sticks in your mind. Chronic pain consumes so much of our attention that it's that much more natural to skip over events and truths that could bring us pain-relieving feelings of joy, happiness, and a sense of safety and security. We skip over information that could tell our alarm system that it's OK to quiet down.

You can learn new skills that counteract these patterns and set yourself on a path to healing and well-being. Savoring is a powerful practice that involves (1) pausing and noticing the sensations (sight, smell, sound, touch, and taste) associated with a pleasant experience as it arises and (2) basking in any positive feelings (joy, contentment, satisfaction, peace) that emerge. Studies suggest that savoring can help improve how well the reward system works and lower pain. I've seen it work firsthand. As a research fellow at Johns Hopkins, part of my job involved lead-ing research volunteers with rheumatoid arthritis though a four-session savoring meditation protocol as part of a trial funded by the National Institutes of Health. Overall, the people I worked with said they enjoyed the practice and found it easy to do. One participant, a social worker who worked with young people, enjoyed savoring so much that she told me she wanted to practice every day and teach it to her own clients right away. More formally, our findings demonstrated that savoring meditation engaged reward system circuits, increased positive emotions in daily life, and lowered experimental pain (a laboratory measure of alarm system sensitivity). In this study each savoring session was only about 20 min-utes. So, encouragingly, it may be that it doesn't take long to start seeing benefits of savoring practice.

Neuropsychologist Dr. Rick Hanson, an expert in savoring and posi-tive neuroplasticity, says that to rewire the brain away from a fixation on the negative and toward an embracing of the positive, we should inten-tionally savor positive experiences for at least 20 to 30 seconds. To give an example, I'm a dog lover. When I spend a few minutes hugging my dog Arnie (named after Arnold Palmer), I can either pause and deeply enjoy his soft fur and appreciate his sweet, big-hearted personality, or my mind can be elsewhere, racing toward an imagined future in which I have too much to do and not enough time, in which I'll fall short and not be OK. The former reduces pain and increases stress-relieving bio-chemicals, whereas the latter sets off my threat-detection alarm (think stress hormones and inflammatory chemicals). For me, and many others, imagined failures and catastrophes are a go-to destination. Savoring not only counteracts the tendency to get lost in this imagined world but also increases positive feelings that produce internal painkillers (opioids).

What should you savor? You don't need anything elaborate or excep-tional. You can savor ordinary experiences like walking outside to get the mail, a kiss on the cheek, a warm cup of tea or coffee, walking barefoot, laughter, a conversation, the sunrise, the stars, inhaling and exhaling, music. When someone expresses love, appreciation, or a compliment, you can pause and soak it in rather than deflecting or discounting it. You can even savor the absence of something difficult (pain in your feet, con-flict, fatigue, a toothache, no longer being in a stressful situation that you may have experienced in the past). You can also savor positive feelings of anticipating something good (feelings of excitement around getting together with a good friend). You can even savor positive memories from your past (this is especially useful if you're in a flare and aren't getting out much or if you're experiencing a period of particularly intense pain and need a tool to manage it in the moment). All around you is evidence that your body is safe and OK. The trick is to train your mind to embrace these truths.

Let's briefly explore this practice. You might start by savoring a sight out your window right now in this moment, or if you happen to be sitting outside, some aspect of nature. Soften your gaze and, in Hanson's words, let the world come to you. Notice patterns of light and shadow, pleasant colors, and shapes. Maybe you notice pleasant sounds or physical sensations right now as well. Gently notice and absorb any feelings of awe, appreciation, or beauty that arise. That's the general framework for savoring.

Here are step-by-step instructions on how to savor the positive:

1. **Choose something to savor.** It could be something that naturally arises in the moment, or you can intentionally choose something to savor for a few minutes (your dog, a nature walk, a song).

2. **Arrive with mindfulness.** Take a deep breath in, followed by a long exhale. Set an intention to gently bring your attention back to the object of savoring when it wanders.

3. **Use your senses.** Contact the object of savoring with as many senses as are available to you. Experience the object of savoring with sight, sound, smell, touch, and taste. Notice patterns of light, shadow, and color. Receive sounds with the whole body, noticing them as they arise and disappear, noticing space between sounds or a quality of silence. Notice what you smell and taste. Notice any pleasant or neutral physical sensations of pressure, warmth, coolness, or movement that arise.

4. **Absorb positive feelings.** Notice, enjoy, and appreciate any positive feelings (calm, peace, joy, awe, gratitude, appreciation, happiness, contentment, interest, serenity) that arise. You might visualize positive feelings sinking into you, like rain into soil. Imagine your body and heart opening to receive what is good about this experience.

5. Notice what feels meaningful. You might find that as you savor, you are reminded of important truths, insights, or memories that are meaningful to you. For instance, perhaps savoring a memory of a joyful family gathering reminds you of how interconnected you are with your ancestors and with future generations. Or maybe you're reminded of how family is the most important thing to you, and of your desire to be more present with your spouse, parents, siblings, or kids. If nothing comes to mind, that's OK. But if something does, include it in your meditation.

I recommend practicing savoring every day for at least five minutes, and the more the better. You can set aside time for formal practice, as well as intentionally savor positive things that happen in your day spontaneously.

A powerful combination is to savor in nature. In Chapter 3 I mentioned the Japanese tradition known as forest bathing (*shinrin-yoku*), which involves slow, long walks in the woods while savoring the awe-inspiring details of the natural world (trees, plants, rocks, streams, sounds of birds, and so much more). Scientific studies have shown that forest bathing increases positive feelings, reduces pain, and improves how well the immune system works. Fascinatingly, when we're in nature, we inhale compounds that plants give off to protect themselves (phytoncides), which can help increase the number of infection- and cancer-fighting cells in our own bodies. Savoring in nature may also promote nondual awareness, or a sense of oneness with the earth, which can promote pain-relieving feelings of calm and peace. I invite you to engage in this practice following these steps:

1. **Choose a natural setting.** You can savor any aspect of nature: a forest, ocean, garden, open field, open sky. You can sit outside on a porch and listen to the rain.

2. **Set an intention.** Mindfully savor your time in nature without distractions, without looking at your phone. Try to set aside at least thirty minutes for this activity (the longer the better, but any amount of time you have available will be of benefit).

3. **Arrive in the present.** Note to yourself, I have arrived. I'm not coming from anywhere, and I'm not on my way somewhere. Right now,

I enjoy and appreciate the earth's natural wonders. I allow myself to be held and nourished by Mother Earth.

4. **Experience nature with the five senses.** Allow yourself to explore and linger near places that you find peaceful or intriguing. Notice physical sensations (the earth beneath your feet, the texture of a tree, the coolness of a stream), sounds (birdsong, the breeze hitting leaves, the silence between sounds), sights (greens, light beams between leaves), smells, and any tastes. Fully absorb the beauty of nature through the doorway of the senses. Allow yourself to become childlike, in awe of this new, mysterious world, one that you've (really!) never seen before. As you become distracted (by thoughts, pain sensations), return your attention to the sensory experience.

5. **Absorb positive emotions.** If any positive emotions arise (peace, awe, appreciation), receive them openly in your body, mind, and spirit. Let them sink into and fill you.

6. **Notice what feels meaningful.** Notice and receive any insights or meanings that arise during this exercise. Perhaps a sense of oneness with the earth or universe arises, and you remember that you're never truly separate or alone. Maybe you notice you're more in touch with your ancestors, spiritual figures, or religious beliefs. Maybe you feel gratitude for the innumerable wonders that Mother Earth offers in each moment.

Remember the key concept: If you don't experience pain relief right away from this exercise, that's OK. Remember, you're retraining your alarm system to incorporate pleasant and safe information into its decision-making process, to ultimately make it less sensitive. Effects on pain intensity aside, the practices presented in this chapter will enrich and deepen your life.

8

Self-Compassion

One of the most consistent sources of suffering I see in my practice is the relentless inner critic. Mean, degrading, and knowing no bounds, it can attack any aspect of our inner life, including the way we manage an illness and even our efforts to be more mindful or peaceful. *You're not taking care of yourself right. Get it together, would you?! You should be meditating and exercising more. What's wrong with you? Why can't you just get motivated! It's your fault you're not feeling well today. I don't know why you're still upset about this. Just get over it.* Although deeply misguided, deep down the inner critic has a benevolent purpose: it thinks, *If I strong-arm this person into shape, maybe they'll be more competent, capable, healthy, and, ultimately, loved.* Yet it leaves us feeling sad and beaten down, and it only sabotages our efforts to take care of ourselves and others effectively. The negative emotions that result from self-criticism (shame, guilt, despair) can make pain worse. Think of self-criticism as a threat, albeit an internal one. We wouldn't speak to our friends the way we do to ourselves in our very wildest dreams.

REFLECT: I invite you to take a moment to reflect on self-critical narratives that might be present in your life. During difficult moments (pain flares, mistakes, conflicts), do you beat yourself up? Do you harshly try to strong-arm yourself into being different in some way? Have you started believing stigmatizing messages about people with chronic pain (that you're not enough, defective, faking it, or a burden)? Or do you encourage yourself with kindness and understanding? What are the familiar voices and feelings that come up during moments of struggle? Write what comes to mind below or in a journal if you like.

....

....

....

Fortunately, there is an antidote to self-criticism: self-compassion. *Self-compassion* is a term coined by pioneering researcher Dr. Kristin Neff, who was influenced by Buddhist psychology and empirically characterized self-compassion and its benefits through a great many scientific studies. Self-compassion has three components: (1) mindfulness (being nonjudgmentally aware of our experience), (2) self-kindness (treating ourselves lovingly), and (3) common humanity (the recognition that we are never alone in our experience, as our struggles, no matter how rare or complicated, are part of being human and others experience them too). In many ways, people who are more self-compassionate tend to fare better than those who are less so. Self-compassion is distinguishable from self-esteem. Self-esteem is a tenuous way of feeling good about ourselves because it rests on how much we accomplish and produce. All in good time each of us loses our ability to produce according to consumer capitalist standards. Does that mean we're no longer lovable? Self-compassion means holding our ever-changing experiences and (dis) abilities with compassion and understanding.

If you notice that you're speaking to yourself harshly and that you react with emotions like shame and self-hatred, self-compassion may be an important tool in your pain care toolbox. You *can* change your inner narratives to be more compassionate, and research suggests that doing so may increase pain-relieving prosocial positive emotions (love, benevolence, kindness, warmth, and forgiveness), reduce pain, and improve quality of life. For example, learning and practicing lovingkindness meditation, an ancient Buddhist practice which involves generating warm and benevolent feelings toward oneself and others, has been shown to help people manage chronic low back pain. It has been shown to help lower pain, anger, and distress in daily life. Lovingkindness meditation is backed by science and involves offering loving wishes in the form of verbal phrases like the following:

> *May I be safe and protected.*
> *May I be filled with deep healing.*
> *May I be happy and at ease.*
> *May I touch great and natural peace.*

These phrases are then offered to friends, acquaintances, people who are difficult or challenging, and eventually, all sentient creatures. Other small trials in people with pain suggest favorable effects of self-compassion on pain and well-being. More broadly, there is strong scientific evidence that self-compassion practices can relieve stress and improve mental health. As a psychologist I view self-compassion as essential. When I'm working with clients, I'm always listening for the self-critical narrative that's getting piled on top of whatever raw pain is being experienced. In my experience when people begin to relate to themselves with more kindness and love, their inner life and outer relationships tend to benefit.

There's a phrase that deeply resonated with me on a meditation retreat I attended several years ago. After hours and hours of sitting meditation practice, I found myself at war with myself and what I was feeling. Frustrated by a distracted mind and physical pain, I wrestled with each experience and with myself like an enemy. One of the teachers suggested that rather than go to war, I simply ask, *Can I meet this life as it's presenting itself to me?* In a flash of insight I realized that my self-criticism was really a way of trying to manage and control life, as opposed to allowing it to unfold with an attitude of acceptance and love. That realization helped me let go, and I felt an immediate sense of emotional relief.

You can start building self-compassion today. There are many different ways to cultivate this vital resource. Let's review a few practices together. I invite you to begin practicing whichever exercises resonate the most with you.

Writing Exercises

REFLECT AND WRITE: If my best friend, a young child or pet, or some-one else I love dearly were experiencing what I've been going through lately, what would I say to them?

. . . .

. . . .

. . . .

REFLECT AND WRITE: If my dearest friends and loved ones (including pets) knew about my internal struggles, what would they say to me?

. . . .

. . . .

. . . .

REFLECT AND WRITE: Imagine your future self, say 10, 15, or 20 years from now. Imagine yourself in the form of a wise, evolved, and under-standing elder. What would your future self want you to know and trust?

. . . .

. . . .

. . . .

Review what you wrote above and try to commit it to memory. Each time you notice yourself going down the path of self-criticism in your daily life, gently offer yourself the messages you wrote above.

Imagery Exercises

Kind Friend Practice

To practice this exercise first read the instructions in their entirety. Then close your eyes if that works for you and practice for 5 to 10 minutes. Bring to mind a kind, wise, loving, and evolved being. It could be a grandmother, friend, religious or spiritual figure, or a line of ancestors. It might be your future self, after you've accumulated years of wisdom and understanding. Pick whatever figure most emanates kindness, love, and acceptance. Take a few moments to allow this figure to join you right here in this moment. Notice how they're filled with joy upon seeing you. You might imagine them sitting next to you, taking you by the hand, filling you, or even taking over the controls inside of you, capable of giving you exactly what you need, ready to respond to your inner life in the most kind, loving, and forgiving way. Let this being's kindness fill you now. Be open to receive their love and compassion and notice if they offer a message. Bask in any feelings of love, kindness, and compassion that may arise.

Inner Child Exercise

Children yearn for love and understanding, but the world cannot provide those things 100 percent of the time. Inside us, metaphorically, we each have an inner child that at times feels afraid, alone, misunderstood, angry, or sad. Unaddressed childhood wounds can have an impact on how we think and feel, even if we're not fully aware of them. The good news is that we can reparent our inner child by offering them our full attention and love. Buddhist monastic Thich Nhat Hanh writes about how important it is to embrace our inner child with tenderness.

I invite you now to take a moment to call to mind the younger you. It could be any age. If you're not sure which to choose, try the six-year-old you. Picture your younger self in your mind's eye as vividly as you can. Notice how that child is feeling and what they may be believing about themselves or the world. Imagine yourself holding them with utmost love, tenderness, and compassion. Let them know that their feelings are valid and understandable. Let them know that they're seen, safe, protected, and loved. See how much tenderness you can offer your inner child now, in this moment. Let them know that you aren't turning your back on them, that you're staying right there with them, no matter what. Offer your inner child your curiosity, interest, and respect. After practicing for a few minutes, when you're ready, bring your attention back to the here and now. Set an intention to pause and offer compassion to your inner child whenever you're feeling upset or overwhelmed.

Daily Life Practices

You can practice self-compassion on the go using three simple steps:

1. **Mindful labeling.** Start by labeling your bodily sensations, thoughts, and feelings. For example, *worry, racing thoughts, planning, analyzing, tightness in the throat and jaw, increasing pain.* This can help prevent you from getting overly caught up in your experience.

2. **Offer self-kindness.** Experiment with thinking something like this: *I'm struggling not because there's something wrong with me, but because this is a hard situation. I offer love and care toward myself.*

3. **Remember common humanity.** At least 20 percent of people around the globe live with chronic pain. You're not bad or defective for having chronic pain, and you're not alone.

I also like to practice **walking lovingkindness.** When I'm in line at the grocery store or driving, for example, I try to remember to offer the lovingkindness phrases (*may you be safe, may you be happy, may you be at ease,* etc.) to others around me. I immediately find that the practice helps me feel calmer and less self-absorbed. This practice is completely opposite of what is essentially considered normal behavior in these situations (being angry about having to wait, criticizing the incompetence of other drivers, or ruminating about one's to-do list). Try this practice to boost your brain's reward system.

Radically experiment with offering kindness **to the pain sensation itself.** Gently note, *I forgive you for being here. May you be at ease. May you be at peace. May you be filled with love and kindness.* This practice counteracts the natural tendency to go to war with the pain.

At the end of the day, remember that

- you don't have to earn love;
- you're allowed to feel things deeply;
- it's OK to say no;
- it's OK to need help;

- it's OK to not feel well;
- it's a strength to be gentle, nurturing, and forgiving toward yourself; and
- you can always begin again. If you go down the old road of self-blame and criticism, hold that too with compassion and start again.

9

Benefiting Others

Now that we've explored self-compassion and the feel-good prosocial emotions that can flow from it, let's turn our attention to prosocial behavior, which is defined as voluntary actions intended to benefit others. Kind and altruistic acts can reduce pain through several pathways. Remember what pain neuroscience tells us: chronic pain is the brain's danger alarm system getting stuck in high gear, and when we're under threat, we naturally become self-focused. Since the pain signal is so attention-grabbing (by design), it's easy for pain to consume most of our finite attentional resources, thus leaving little "brainpower" for doing things that might produce pain-relieving positive emotions and counteract a narrowed, pain-focused attentional state. Prosocial activity is a direct antidote to self-focused worry and physical inactivity that pain tends to promote. It expands our attention beyond the pain and worry, imbues our life with meaning and purpose, and promotes physical activity and engagement with life. Acts of kindness and generosity can create a "helper's high" or "warm glow" sensation along with feelings of love, joy, accomplishment, and competence, which is the reward system at work.

Well-controlled experiments and studies that have been done out in the "real world" show that prosocial activity can lower pain, enhance the reward system, and protect our bodies from the effects of stress. Experimentally induced prosocial behaviors like charitable giving, affectionate communication, and acting kindly toward others have been shown to increase pain-lowering feelings of happiness as well as reduce stress-induced cortisol (the "stress hormone") production. Providing help and support in real-world settings protects people from the physical and mental health consequences of stress, reduces interpersonal conflict, increases how much social support people receive, and enhances life satisfaction and self-esteem. Providing help and care can increase *social capital*, a term that refers to the number and quality of social relationships people have. When we act kindly, others in our social network are likely to reciprocate. As discussed earlier healthy social bonds are a crucial part of any pain relief journey. They are an enduring source of pain-relieving positive emotions and experiences (for instance, laughing with other people has been shown to promote the release of our body's natural painkillers). In sum prosocial behavior is an important tool in your pain care toolbox that can help dampen how loud your pain alarm is.

Jeffrey, an older adult, took advantage of benefiting others as a pain coping tool. He volunteered at the local library a few hours each week. He would tell me how much it helped him get out of his own head, meet new people, feel gratified about contributing to others, and get active. As Jeffrey shows, there are multiple healing mechanisms at play when you get out and help others.

There are innumerable ways to serve others. Helping can be formal (such as through volunteer work with an organization), or more informal (spontaneous kind acts for someone else). You can give time, money, or possessions. One type of prosociality that's long been of interest to scientists working within the positive psychology tradition (the science and practice of nurturing human strengths as opposed to simply reducing mental distress) is prosocial behavior expressed through *random acts of kindness*. These are small acts that we do that can be immediately rewarding, that are out of the ordinary, and that take only a little bit of extra effort. Research suggests that a few acts of kindness per day over a period of days or weeks can promote positive feelings (a sign of the reward system working well) and reduce mental distress. Related research suggests that the more variety you build into your acts of kindness the better, because the reward system likes novelty. You can perform random acts of kindness for friends, strangers, family, animals, and the planet as a whole.

REFLECT: Take a moment and brainstorm random acts of kindness that you could perform over the next week. Try to think of things that are small and easily doable. Examples include taking out an elderly neighbor's trash; being patient and kind toward every service professional you interact with; picking up litter; reducing, reusing, and recycling; or calling friends on their birthday. Feel free to jot down any ideas here or in a journal:

....

....

....

I've listed some suggested random acts of kindness below. Feel free to check off any ideas that you like. Try a random act of kindness challenge. This week, commit to two to five random acts of kindness per day over seven days to both boost your reward system and spread kindness in our world.

- ❑ Write kind and encouraging words on sticky notes and leave them around the house or in your family members' lunch boxes.
- ❑ Make your spouse a cup of tea or coffee or cook their favorite meal.
- ❑ Write to people in your life who may be lonely.
- ❑ Send cards for various occasions: birthdays, anniversaries, and graduations.
- ❑ Make a meal or cookies for an elderly neighbor.
- ❑ At the store let people go ahead of you in line.
- ❑ When driving let other cars pass you.
- ❑ Try to compliment as many people in a day as you can.

❑ Give each person you're speaking with your full presence and attention.

❑ Send sympathy, encouragement, or "get well soon" cards.

❑ Smile, make eye contact, and thank every worker you interact with (cashiers, retail workers).

❑ If you have the energy, do a little extra around the house.

❑ Send friends or family members a letter of gratitude telling them how much you love and appreciate them. It might feel awkward or vulnerable to do this, but it's a science-backed practice that can make an impact.

❑ When you feel proud of someone, tell them.

❑ Write positive comments on others' social media posts. More generally, vow to only write positive material online.

❑ Smile and say good morning to everyone you pass.

❑ If you own property, plant a tree. Your whole neighborhood will benefit.

❑ Hand out water bottles to people working outside in the heat.

❑ Leave water or snacks outside your door for delivery workers.

❑ Smile and thank the people who collect your trash and recycling.

❑ Write great reviews and fill out customer satisfaction surveys when you're happy with the help you received.

❑ Mindfully donate your stuff. For instance, donate books to a local library. As you do so, appreciate the kind gesture that you're making and imagine other people benefiting from this kind act.

❑ Buy or donate a sleeping bag and tent to an unhoused individual.

❑ At work, take in snacks to share. When coworkers contribute or do well on something, compliment and uplift them in front of other colleagues.

❑ Text friends that you think may be going through a hard time. Reach out to old friends. Share pictures and updates about your life.

❑ Help out new parents by bringing them dinner and offer to watch the baby while they eat and relax.

❑ Fill up a jar with "reasons I love you" notes and give it to someone you love.

❑ Tip generously when you can.

❑ Donate money (even small amounts) to causes you care about.

❑ Learn about diverse cultures.

❑ Use reusable bags on all shopping trips.

❑ Find new uses for old things around the house.

❑ Shop at a local farmers' market.

❑ Take three deep breaths before responding to someone who is irritating you.

❑ Write a thank-you note to your mail carrier.

Volunteering

Volunteering can boost the reward system despite being more time consuming than random acts of kindness. Volunteering can enhance pain-relieving resources like social connection, physical activity, and positive feelings. If you have time consider getting involved in your community. Hospitals, farms, public parks and gardens, art/theater centers, and animal shelters are just a few examples of places that are often seeking volunteers. Think about things that might be fun and interesting to you. On the AARP's Create the Good website (*https://createthegood.aarp.org*) you can fill out a volunteer interest form and receive suggested opportunities based on your unique interests. You can search for opportunities in your area or online at *https://volunteermatch.org*. It may sound exhausting, but remember, getting active and giving your brain opportunities to experience rewards (and other-focused activity may be more rewarding than self-focused activity) *is* pain treatment. Be gentle with yourself and try to commit to a volunteer activity that feels manageable and not overwhelming.

Chronic Pain Advocacy

Another way of serving others is to use your expertise and understanding as someone living with chronic pain to benefit other people experiencing the same. There is research suggesting that people with pain who give back to others with pain see personal benefits. If this might be of interest to you, I recommend exploring the wonderful volunteer resources available through the U.S. Pain Foundation, a reputable patient advocacy group. For instance, with their support and training you can start your own peer-led chronic pain support group. You can submit articles to *Remedy* (*https://uspainfoundation.org/news/blog*), a blog that publishes patient stories, perspectives, advice, and recommendations designed to help others living with pain. You can learn how to volunteer for research studies (including surveys that you can easily do from your couch), learn how to take action on pain policy and meet with your legislators to discuss pain issues, set up fundraisers for pain care (in person and online), host an information booth about chronic pain care at your local library or community center, and more. You can make a difference. Start here: *https://uspainfoundation.org/volunteer.*

Overarching Mindset Strategies

Here are a few general mindset strategies to bear in mind as you increase prosocial activity as part of your pain care plan:

• Approach kind acts with a process-oriented mindset and let go of attachment to any outcome. While acts of kindness can boost your reward system, paradoxically holding onto that as the goal and stressing out if you don't see results right away can steal the joy of giving.

• We do things every day to support other people that can feel obligatory (laundry, yard work, caregiving, going to work each day). Try replacing "have to" with "get to" to shift your mindset. Validate yourself for everything you do ("Today I signed my kid up for dance lessons, gave my partner an extra hug, and called my grandmother. All that matters. I made a difference today.").

• In every interaction, prioritize being kind over being right. This mindset will promote more rewarding interactions and make conversations more fruitful.

• If you don't have the energy to do prosocial activities, that's OK. Listen to your intuition about what feels manageable to you and try to challenge yourself bit by bit.

10

Pursuing Meaning in Life

I s it possible to lead a meaningful life with chronic pain? This is an important question that I imagine you've considered deeply and often. Chronic pain can feel devastating, torturous, unrelenting, and monstrous. It can put a knife in meaningful pursuits that once offered aim and purpose. You might feel like you've lost important parts of your identity. At the same time, research suggests that those who feel that life remains meaningful despite persistent pain tend to fare better (reduced pain and increased well-being) than those who start to feel like their life is meaningless.

Having meaning and purpose has been viewed by some as essential for transcending suffering in horrific circumstances. Through his observations of prisoners in Nazi concentration camps, psychiatrist Victor Frankl inferred that what he termed the *will to meaning*, or the basic human desire to find and realize meaning and purpose, helped people existing within a mass genocide maintain the will to live. Indeed, psychological science has supported the position that seeing aspects of our lives as meaningful and significant can help see us through hardship.

I view meaning making as a way of stopping the war with pain and opening up new opportunities to boost the reward system. If the pain won't go away, at least for now, you can still sow the seeds of a life that is of benefit to this precious planet and to those around you. Focusing on living a meaningful life with chronic pain coming along for the ride (as opposed to waiting for the pain to go away) may just open up opportunities for positive emotions, social connections, and other resilience resources.

Finding Purpose

How can you cultivate meaning and purpose? One way is to follow the principles of acceptance and commitment therapy (ACT), an evidence-based treatment for chronic pain (and several other conditions). The basic idea behind ACT is that we can take our unpleasant thoughts, feelings, and sensations with us (*accept* that they're there) while we continue to do (*commit to*) things we value. This involves being clear about what you value in life and then identifying actions that keep you in line with those values as best you can. Conceptually, you need to be courageously willing to have the experiences that show up while staying committed to what you value most. Values are like a compass. They help keep us on course through the joys and sorrows of this life. Using mindfulness (nonjudgmental, kind awareness of our experience), we can continually notice when we've fallen off course and reorient our actions toward our values.

REFLECT: I invite you to reflect for a moment on your values. What matters most to you? What do you stand for? How do you aspire to treat others? What personal qualities do you like to embody? What do you want to leave behind for future generations? Looking back on your life, what do you want to be able to say about how you lived it? Write what comes to mind below or in a journal or simply reflect on these prompts.

....

....

....

To support your reflection, you can review the list of common values in the box on the next page and circle or highlight those that feel most important to you.

COMMON VALUES

acceptance, accomplishment, adventurousness, altruism, appreciating the sacred, appreciation of diversity, art appreciation, attentiveness, authenticity, balance, beauty, belonging, benevolence, bravery, cheerfulness, cleanliness, collaboration, commitment, communication, community, compassion, competence, concentration, concern for others, connection, contemplative practice (prayer, meditation), cooperation, courage, creativity, culture, decisiveness, determination, discovery, empathy, encouragement, energy, enjoyment, enthusiasm, environmental stewardship, equality, excellence, fairness, faith, family, flexibility, forgiveness, freedom, friendship, fun, generosity, gentleness, good health, goodwill, gratitude, healthy boundaries, humility, humor, independence, inner peace, innovation, integrity, intelligence, interdependence, intimacy, joy, justice, kindness, knowledge, leadership, letting go, lifelong learning, living in the present, love, loyalty, meaning, mindfulness, nature connection, nonviolence, oneness/self-transcendence, openness to others' viewpoints, patience, peace, perseverance, personal growth, physical fitness, pleasure, practicality, prosperity, reconciliation, reliability, religion, resourcefulness, respect for others, responsiveness, safety, security, self-control, serenity, service, simplicity, spirituality, strength, success, teamwork, tolerance, tradition, tranquility, trust, truthfulness, vitality, wisdom

Aligning Values and Actions

Every day we do things that keep us in line with our values and things that take us away from them. For example, I really value living in the present. Doing a morning meditation session keeps me aligned with that value, while skipping my practice to get more done or avoid unpleasant feelings moves me away. I value maintaining good health as long as I can. Getting up for a 10-minute walk or to do a few yoga poses every hour supports that, whereas sitting for four-hour stretches in a slouched position does not.

Be wary of pain management strategies taking over your life. To illustrate, let's say Joe, who lives with chronic pain, circled *family* as one of his primary values. Meanwhile, acupuncture is a treatment that he knows helps lower his pain. He starts skipping his kids' choir concerts to go to acupuncture appointments twice a week. In so doing, Joe is preventing his brain and body from experiencing the positive emotions and meaning that would come from actions (attending the concerts) that are in line with his values (family). Remember this principle: You need to balance doing pain treatments that you know lower your pain with living your life because staying actively involved in things that matter to you *is* treatment. It promotes a sense of meaning and purpose, which can help you stay resilient in the face of chronic pain. It opens up opportunities to experience reward, which can lower pain. Regardless of how doing valued activities impacts your pain intensity, you can take stock of your life and say that you're still doing things that matter.

EXERCISE

As a reflection exercise I invite you to choose three values from the box on the previous page and reflect on how (mis)aligned your actions have been with those values over the past month.

Value: ....

Aligned actions: ....

Misaligned actions: ....

Value: ....

Aligned actions: ....

Misaligned actions: ....

Value: ....

Aligned actions: ....

Misaligned actions: ....

I now invite you to come up with three achievable, action-oriented goals to try over the next two weeks that will help you act in line with your values. For example, if you value nature connection, you might set a goal to plant one small plant in a pot. Things like that. One day and one small thing at a time. You can do this!

Short-term goals:

1. ....

2. ....

3. ....

Reflecting on your short-term goals, now set three longer-term goals to try to achieve over the next six months. Continuing with the nature connection value, you might set a goal to plant and care for a vegetable garden this spring with five different plants.

Long-term goals:

1. ....

2. ....

3. ....

Come back and revisit your goals often. If you fall off course, simply start again. You might find it helpful to share your goals with a friend or family member.

Staying Flexible and Honoring Your Feelings

Thinking about ways to maintain meaning and purpose in your life when you have chronic pain might bring about grief and sadness. It's OK to grieve the things you've lost, like your seemingly endless energy, mental clarity, and ease of living. Many people with chronic pain and illness describe the need to adjust to a new normal. I'm not suggesting that you simply go back to doing everything you loved and valued at 100 percent intensity before your chronic pain started. I'm advocating for flexibility and creativity as you (re)consider old and new ways of nurturing meaning and purpose in your life. You can hold grief and hope at the same time. Honor all feelings that arise as you set meaningful and realistic goals that are best suited to your current circumstances. Trust that engagement in valued activities is boosting your brain's reward system and keeping you on the path to better health.

How Have You Grown?

It may sound trite, but don't forget to congratulate yourself on the ways that you've withstood the horror of chronic pain and even grown through it in some ways. Are you more compassionate, understanding, loving, accepting, strong, resourceful, flexible, or determined? Have you learned things about yourself or others? Pause and appreciate any strengths that come to mind now in this moment.

PART FOUR

LOWERING INFLAMMATION TO HEAL CHRONIC PAIN

Inflammation is an important part of your body's danger response system. When you come down with the flu or a cold, your body immediately orchestrates an elaborate response that attacks and eliminates the harmful invading virus. It does the same when you catch strep throat, and the invaders are bacteria. Thanks to inflammation the body survives and thrives after infection. Inflammation is also set off by extreme heat or cold, mechanical forces (getting injured in a car accident for instance), and chemicals (environmental irritants ranging from indoor and outdoor pollution, high alcohol consumption, and smoking to proinflammatory chemicals found in plastics, cleaning products, fragrances, and cosmetics).

Unfortunately, inflammation can get stuck in persistent, chronic overdrive. When this occurs, inflammation no longer fights disease but rather contributes to it. Chronic inflammation fosters chronic pain as well as a host of other diseases (diabetes, cancer, cardiovascular disease, Alzheimer's disease, depression, etc.). Chronic inflammation contributes to symptoms of painful conditions like rheumatoid arthritis and inflammatory bowel disease and is also observed in chronic low back pain, temporomandibular disorder, chronic migraine, chronic neck pain, and numerous other pain conditions.

Chronic inflammation and chronic pain often go hand in hand. Inflammation stimulates the body's danger receptors. Danger receptors then communicate a threat alert to the brain, increasing the likelihood that pain will be experienced.

The immune system is incredibly complex, and scientists are actively trying to understand its many moving parts and identify new treatment approaches to address chronic inflammation. We do, however, already have abundant scientific evidence that chronic inflammation (and therefore pain) can be reduced substantially by addressing poor diet, inadequate sleep, and physical inactivity—an interrelated trifecta of threats that activate the inflammatory branch of the alarm system. Here's how it can work: Poor sleep tends to increase the chance we'll reach for junk food, which further saps our energy and compounds the likelihood we'll avoid exercise and spend the day on the couch. That's why improving one of these areas has the potential to favorably affect the others.

Chronic stress is another major contributor to inflammation, and you've been reading about how to tackle stress throughout this book—by reducing threats ramping up your alarm system and by increasing positive emotions, which can relieve stress. As noted above, one other factor causes inflammation—environmental irritants. This is an enormous topic and the subject of entire books, but Chapter 13 offers some targeted recommendations.

11

Eat to Live
Lower Inflammation with Food

One of the most powerful tools available to reduce pain-exacerbating systemic inflammation is a healthy diet. If this comes as a surprise know that nutrition therapy only came into the spotlight within the past 5 to 10 years as chronic pain treatment. Nutrition therapy is broadly defined as any professionally prescribed diet and may include specific nutrients, antioxidants, or supplements (pre- or probiotics, omega-3 fatty acids, vitamins, or minerals) designed to benefit health. Leading pain research organizations advocate for optimizing diet as part of multidisciplinary pain treatment because research shows that nutrition therapies have pain-relieving effects. In simple survey studies, where people describe their dietary habits and pain scores, those with healthier diets report lower pain.

Symptoms of several common chronic pain conditions are associated with nutrition, including osteoarthritis, rheumatoid arthritis, fibromyalgia, back pain, irritable bowel syndrome, pelvic pain (such as from endometriosis), diabetic neuropathy, migraine, postherpetic neuralgia, and carpal tunnel syndrome. Yes, even pain felt in just one area of the body such as the back or wrist can be impacted by how and what we eat. Therefore, experts argue that a comprehensive nutrition evaluation and treatment plan led by a dietitian should be included in every pain management program.

Gut Health and Chronic Pain

If you've been noticing an abundance of news about gut health, you've probably run across the term *microbiome*. How the microbiome is connected to inflammation and chronic illness (and pain) is one of the most fascinating frontiers in research today. The microbiome is the mass of bacteria, viruses, fungi, and parasites that live in and on the body. Microbial cells (like bacteria) in the microbiome outnumber human cells. This fascinating fact challenges the very notion of who "we" are! We think our body is "ours," yet perhaps this is inaccurate. In fact, "we" are an entire community! Whether and how our body deploys an inflammatory response in a particular moment is directly impacted by our microbiome, which is predominately located in our stomach, intestines, and colon (the gut).

There are so many fascinating reasons to take excellent care of the gut to protect our health. Most of the immune system, which controls inflammation, is in the gut lining, and so what we put into our bodies really can stimulate or curb inflammation. Further, there are about 100 million neurons in the gut, which are collectively known as the enteric nervous system. Researchers have nicknamed the enteric nervous system the "second brain." You can think about it this way: basically, you have two "brains"—one in your gut and one in your head—and they communicate constantly. The brain in your gut, just like the brain in your head, releases several neurochemicals associated with mood and pain relief, including opioids, glutamate, serotonin, and dopamine. So we're continuing to discover in fascinating ways how gut feelings are in fact "real." Several disorders are associated with changes in the microbiome, including fibromyalgia and depression.

The baseline takeaway here is that your gut and microbiome are incredibly precious to your very existence, not to mention your physical and mental health. Reflecting on this truth may help you find the motivation to make needed but difficult changes in your life. For more on this topic see Dr. Emeran Mayer's acclaimed book, *The Mind-Gut Connection: How the Hidden Conversation Within Our Bodies Impacts Our Mood, Our Choices, and Our Overall Health.*

Let's look at the downside of the gut-pain equation: some of the foods we eat can promote inflammation. If you haven't come across it yet, the term *ultra-processed* is worth knowing. Ultra-processed foods are those that have been dramatically changed from their original state. For instance, frozen chicken nuggets with added sodium, preservatives, and artificial colors are the ultra-processed version of the whole, unaltered original: chicken. A frozen apple pie with added sugars and dyes is an ultra-processed version of apples. Other examples of ultra-processed foods include soda, candy, pizza, chips, shelf-stable breads, sugary cereals, and whipped topping, to name just a few. Ultra-processed foods are typically low in fiber, protein, and nutrients.

Research shows that ultra-processed foods significantly increase inflammation. When these foods enter the body, the alarm system ramps up: *danger!* Think of ultra-processed foods like a roadblock on the road to chronic pain recovery. They also increase your risk of other life-altering health problems like cardiovascular disease. Ultra-processed food manufacturing and consumption is extremely common in North America, which can make it feel like these foods are harmless. Don't be fooled.

Importantly, not everything that comes in a package is ultra-processed. Many foods have been altered only a little bit and are part of a healthy diet: think canned beans or tuna, tofu, hummus, or fresh breads, basic pasta sauce, yogurts, and cheeses that have just a few ingredients and no added sugar. As a general principle things that come in a package that have just a handful of easily recognizable ingredients are considered "processed" as opposed to ultra-processed.

Fortunately, unprocessed and some processed foods are like "green lights" that can make the road to chronic pain recovery quicker and easier. They are a cornerstone of an anti-inflammatory diet, which is recommended in chronic pain management. Let's take a closer look.

The Anti-Inflammatory Diet

Nutrition therapy had profound effects on my own pain problem. I finally met a doctor who conceptualized personalized nutrition as first-line treatment and helped me adopt a whole-food, anti-inflammatory, additive-free diet. She recommended I adopt a high-vegetable elimination diet free from certain food groups that could be acting as hidden food triggers (dairy, gluten, soy, nuts), food additives, and processed foods for 90 days, without "cheating." She also recommended targeted supplements including magnesium, vitamin B_{12}, omega-3s, and probiotics. I then reintroduced foods I had eliminated one by one, to assess whether I had any hidden food sensitivities causing inflammation and pain. The diet helped bring my body back into balance, and the reduction in my pain was so dramatic that I maintain an anti-inflammatory, whole-food diet to this day (albeit less restrictive than my initial elimination diet). Prior to doing systematic nutrition therapy, I played around with cutting out gluten for a week or two here, dairy for a few days there, and eliminated caffeine. Nothing worked, and I erroneously concluded that food had no effect on my pain. Ha! When I worked with a nutrition expert and stuck to the plan consistently for months, everything changed.

If you haven't yet come across a health professional recommending systematic dietary evaluation and treatment, it doesn't mean that diet change isn't potentially very important for you. It just reflects how mainstream clinical treatment for chronic pain is only slowly adopting the recommendations to include nutrition therapy as part of a multidisciplinary pain treatment plan. It's also an indication of the fractured nature of our health-care system, where it's usually up to the patient to identify and reach out to various providers to curate a multimodal care program. Further, as the volume of high-quality, randomized controlled trials on nutrition interventions for chronic pain continues to rise, I imagine (and hope) that nutrition therapy for chronic pain will be fully integrated into pain care.

So, can you land on an anti-inflammatory diet to ease your chronic pain? Before we dive into the dietary guidelines that are generally recommended for chronic pain, here are a few points to keep in mind:

- Identifying the best diets for different pain conditions is an active area of research, so watch for new findings as time goes on.

- Different types of diets, like plant-based diets and Mediterranean diets, have been shown to help pain. When we identify the elements they have in common, such as eating whole foods, increasing fruits and vegetables, and forgoing ultra-processed foods, we'll have important information about what matters.

- Adopting commonly recognized dietary recommendations for

general good health and for chronic pain is good, but getting a personal-ized dietary evaluation and plan can be even better. Each person and chronic pain situation is unique. If you have chronic low back pain, are prediabetic, and want to improve your metabolic health, your plan may be quite different from a person with gastrointestinal symptoms plus chronic migraine and certain food sensitivities or intolerances.

Research shows that patients with pain who do work with a dieti-tian tend to find the process helpful. A nutrition expert can assess your unique situation and collaboratively guide you to the best eating plan for you. They can also provide accountability, periodically assess how well the nutrition plan is working for you, and make any needed adjustments.

General Dietary Recommendations for Lowering Chronic Pain and Inflammation

Following is a summary of recommendations stemming from systematic reviews conducted within the past 5 to 10 years on pain and nutrition, informational products put forth by leading pain research associations, and well-established information about foods that help keep inflamma-tion in check. Consult with your care team as you consider making any dietary changes. *Note: this section is for educational purposes only and does not constitute personalized guidance.*

• **Consider a Mediterranean-style diet.** High in vegetables (including leafy greens), whole fruits, healthy omega-3 fats (found in fish, walnuts, olive oil), legumes (beans, chickpeas, lentils), whole grains, and nuts and seeds, this diet is less likely to cause inflammation than the standard diet of most Americans, which the body interprets as threat-ening, responding with inflammation. The Mediterranean diet includes moderate amounts of cheese and yogurt and little to no red meat, sweets, sugary drinks, or butter consumption. The standard diet in the United States involves ultra-processed and refined starches and meats with pre-servatives.

• **Eat the rainbow.** Add colorful vegetables and fruits to your plate on a regular basis. Fruits (especially berries) and vegetables contain compounds that combat inflammation and oxidative stress. Eat a wide variety of fruits and vegetables each day to "dose" yourself with these anti-inflammatory compounds.

● **Reduce sugar.** Avoid soda and fruit juices as well as other sugary foods (added sugars increase inflammation) such as cakes, cookies, and candy, particularly commercially produced products.

● **Reduce saturated fats and trans fats.** Butter, fatty meats, and high-fat cheese, as well as ultra-processed foods (battered and fried foods, margarine, commercially baked cakes and cookies) should be avoided.

● **Eat only lean animal products.** Namely fish, poultry, and low-fat dairy.

● **Eat whole foods.** Shift away from eating ultra-processed foods to foods in their original, unaltered form: think fresh avocados, vegetables, fruits, fish, and nuts. The body is less likely to think that whole foods (as opposed to boxed crackers and cured meats) are invaders to be dealt with via inflammation.

● **Eliminate food additives.** If you're eating whole foods you'll easily steer clear of added chemicals that give products a longer shelf life.

● **Avoid refined grains.** Favor whole grains (those that look the way they do when pulled out of the ground, like whole millet; barley; teff; amaranth; quinoa; buckwheat; red, black, or brown rice; and sorghum) over ultra-processed cereals, white breads, and white pastas.

● **Maintain an adequate fluid intake.** Dehydration can make pain worse.

● **Increase fiber intake.** Fiber is plentiful in fruits and vegetables as well as whole grains.

● **Avoid caffeine after noon and alcohol.** They impair sleep quality.

● **Consider dietary supplements as advised by a medical provider.** Magnesium, omega-3 fats, vitamin B_{12}, and vitamin D may be useful in some cases.

● **Add omega-3 fats.** Your body doesn't make these anti-inflammatory fats, which are essential for controlling the inflammatory response that our body deploys in response to insults (injury, a virus). Get them from food or supplements: oily fish (salmon, sardines), walnuts, seeds such as flax or chia seeds, and algae.

Change Strategies

Changing your diet, if you decide to do so, can be a huge lift, especially when you're often not feeling well. Here are some behavioral change strategies backed by science:

- **Try to make it a household affair.** Everyone can benefit from a healthy diet! Social support is key. I've noticed my clients have great success when their spouse or family members also decide to improve their diet.

- **Try to make the healthy food choices you make as rewarding as possible.** Practice savoring as you eat something you like: try to fully notice and enjoy the flavors, smells, and textures. Put your fork down after every bite.

- **Try to boost social connection by sharing meals.** Avoid distractions like your phone!

- **Plan ahead.** Cook in bulk over the weekend or prepare vegetables ahead of time and throw them into the fridge.

- **Keep it simple and do what works for you.** I've had a lot of success with roasting or steaming large quantities of vegetables, including frozen ones. It's not fancy, but it works for me.

- **Give up the good for the great.** Tasty fast food feels good, but feeling better feels great.

- **Get personalized guidance.** I believe this is a significant help, but it may not be easy for all; see the next section. In the United States find a credentialed nutrition expert at the Academy of Nutrition and Dietetics' database, *www.eatright.org/find-a-nutrition-expert*.

- **Use self-compassion skills (see Chapter 8) when you find yourself straying from your goals.** The more you can encourage yourself with friendliness, the more likely you are to succeed.

When You Don't Have Time or Money

Pain can make it very hard to have the resources (money, energy, and time) to cook healthy meals. Check out the website No Money No Time (*https://nomoneynotime.com.au*), built by nutrition researchers at the University of Newcastle (no fad diets!). You can filter recipes by what you eat (omnivore or vegetarian, for instance) and cooking equipment you have available. It has a healthy eating quiz you can take as well.

REFLECT AND SET GOALS: As we bring this chapter to a close, take a moment to reflect on how you feel about dietary change. What feels feasible? Where's a good place to start? Are any goals coming to mind? If so, write them below or in a journal:

Goals:

This week: ....

....

This month: ....

....

Over the next six months: ....

....

Barriers:

My biggest barriers to change: ....

....

Strategies I might use to overcome barriers: ....

....

12

Quiet the Alarm and Boost
the Reward System with Good Sleep

We spend a quarter to a third of our lives asleep. Why do we sleep? Fascinatingly, the definitive answer to this question continues to elude us. However, we can say with certainty that good sleep is absolutely critical for our health and functioning, on par (at least!) with nutrition and physical activity. Almost every bodily system is impacted by sleep, and we know that sleep is critical for healthy immune function (including inflammation!) and the functioning of many other systems, including the brain's reward system and our cardiovascular system. Despite the body's being inactive and seemingly at rest, our brains are incredibly active while we're asleep, engaging in life-supporting and "housekeeping" tasks like processing and consolidating information so that we can effectively use it in the future. Sleep also plays a role in removing toxins in the brain that have accumulated during waking hours. Think of sleep as a key time when our brains and bodies restore, reenergize, and repair. Untreated, persistent sleep problems can lead to poorer quality of life and increased risk of chronic pain, as well as heart disease, diabetes, substance use, and other mental health disorders. Value your sleep the same way you do eating, breathing, and socializing: it is essential to being human.

What about sleep and pain? As you've probably experienced, pain can make it harder to sleep, and poor sleep can make pain worse. Poor sleep, which can take many forms, including sleeping for too few hours, waking up a lot in the night, failing to feel rested after sleeping, and more, activates our alarm system. Feeling fatigued, anxious or sad, joyless, overwhelmed, mentally sluggish, and in increased pain reflects what's going on in the body after poor sleep: our alarm system and stress biochemistry (think inflammation, stress hormones like cortisol, and the fight-or-flight response) get ramped up, while our tendency to experience positive emotions (reward system function) goes down. It sets us up to feel pain and enjoy life less.

Scientists are continuing to disentangle precisely how sleep, pain, the reward system, and inflammation interrelate and what it means for better pain treatment. For instance, a 2021 analysis I led at Johns Hopkins, along with our colleagues at UCLA, found that inducing severely disturbed sleep led to more inflammation in the morning than after undisturbed sleep. Interestingly, this was true only in people who reported tending to have fewer positive feelings in daily life, meaning they had poorer reward system functioning. Findings like these point to the potential benefits of improving both sleep and positive emotions to turn down the volume on the alarm system. For example, using the strategies in this chapter combined with the reward system-boosting techniques already introduced could potentially lower your pain.

Simple DIY Strategies for Better Sleep

Here are strategies that can promote good sleep that you can try right away. As you read consider which strategies you're already using and which ones might be worth considering.

- **Be vigilant about your light exposure.** Light is one of the most important factors in regulating your circadian rhythm, which is your internal "clock" that regulates bodily functions, including sleep, according to a 24-hour cycle:
    - *Keep your bedroom as dark as possible.* Consider using blackout curtains or an eye mask to block any artificial light from the street.
    - *Stop looking at blue light (think smartphones) at least an hour before bed.* Blue light, and sometimes green, is activating and has the

same wavelength as the midday sun, so it can trick your body into thinking it's daytime and that you should stay awake. Research has shown, for example, that reading a light-emitting e-book before bed (versus a physical book) makes it take longer to fall asleep and disrupts the internal circadian clock. There is very little scientific evidence backing the effectiveness of products purported to block blue light (blue light-blocking glasses, the iPhone's night shift mode). More broadly, your smartphone provides a sleep degrading trifecta: (1) It offers stimulating content that promotes wakefulness rather than sleepiness (social media feeds, scary news stories). (2) The act of using it for 20 minutes or so (or more!) robs you of time you could be sleeping. (3) As we've reviewed, blue light makes your body think it's daytime. Smartphones are addictive by design, so consider leaving your phone out of the bedroom altogether. Remember, each time you pick it up, someone else is profiting from your lost sleep!

   o *Consider developing a calming ritual before bed that reduces light exposure.* Try deep breathing, meditation, or other spiritual activity with your eyes closed, or read a physical book or magazine. Consider switching from ceiling lights to dim lamps in the evening hours throughout your home.

Sleep experts suggest that getting exposure to sunlight as soon as you wake up in the morning, ideally when the sun is between 10 and 30 degrees above the horizon, can assist in aligning your circadian rhythm, ultimately leading to an improved sleep-wake cycle.

   • **Address racing thoughts.** Many people struggle with a racing mind before bed. If this is you, try these tips:

   o *Keep a journal by your bed and jot down any racing thoughts about "to-do" items.* You can allow yourself to pick them up the next day. After doing so try writing down three things you are grateful for in your life or from the day. This will encourage you to shift out of a fear-based mindset and feel reminded of the ways in which you are safe and already have enough.

   o *Practice mindfulness, prayer or contemplation, or deep breathing for relaxation.* A simple deep breathing practice is to inhale for four counts and exhale for eight. The longer exhale will help your body get into a more relaxed state.

- *Keep the bedroom cool (experts often recommend 65 to 68 degrees Fahrenheit) and as quiet as possible.*

- *Stay active during the day.* Physical activity and exercise will promote tiredness later in the day and get you ready for sleep.

- *Avoid large meals close to bedtime.* Refraining from eating two hours before bed might be a realistic goal.

- *Avoid caffeine after noon.* Drinking it later in the day can keep you up at night.

- *Avoid drinking alcohol and using nicotine.* Although a "nightcap" may seem to help you fall asleep faster, research shows that it disrupts sleep and prevents your brain from entering deep sleep, particularly in the latter part of your sleep window.

- **Keep your bed associated with relaxation and sleep.**

  o *Don't take screens, work, or other stimulating activity into bed.* Keep your bed reserved for sleep and physical intimacy.

  o *Don't try to force yourself to fall asleep.* If you haven't fallen asleep after 20 or 30 minutes, experts say to get out of bed and do something else—meditate, listen to a calming podcast, read a physical book—no screen time. When you start to feel somewhat sleepy, return to bed. If you stay in bed tossing and turning for hours, you will start to associate your bed with stress and wakefulness.

  o *Try to invest in comfortable bedding and a peaceful-feeling, clutter-free bedroom.*

- **Establish a bedtime routine.** Use trial and error, if you haven't already, to determine your best sleeping hours. Are you a night owl, a morning lark, or somewhere in between? Keep consistent bedtimes and wake times, even on the weekends.

Cognitive Behavioral Therapy for Insomnia

Sometimes you might need more than the DIY strategies listed above to see an improvement in sleep. Don't be afraid to seek professional help if you're concerned about your sleep. Start with a primary care doctor or other trusted member of your care team, like a pain specialist. Describe your symptoms, including the impact you're feeling on your quality of life (trouble focusing, daytime sleepiness, and others). Ask if cognitive behavioral therapy for insomnia (CBT-I) may be right for you. CBT-I is considered a first-line treatment for chronic insomnia. It teaches you how to retrain your sleep cycle and deal with stressful nighttime insomnia. It involves identifying and changing the thoughts, feelings, and behaviors that are contributing to sleep problems. Also involved are relaxation training, time-in-bed restriction (reducing the time spent in bed and subsequently increasing it gradually so you spend less time lying in bed awake at night—challenging but highly effective), and managing your environment to make it most conducive to sleep. You can also go directly to the Society of Behavioral Sleep Medicine's website (*https://behavior-alsleep.org*), and explore their provider directory, or search "insomnia specialists" in any of the therapist directories available such as *Psychology Today*'s. CBT-I can be done over telehealth, so it wouldn't necessarily require you to attend in-person appointments.

It's possible to access content that would be taught in CBT-I through a smartphone app, which can be a less expensive option. One option that I would consider reputable and accessible is CBT-i Coach, developed by the U.S. Department of Veterans Affairs.

As a final note, social inequities make it harder for many to get the high-quality sleep they need. Neighborhood noise pollution, light pollution, and air pollution are fundamental problems that can make sleep worse. I don't want to make it sound like doing the simple strategies presented in this chapter can erase the effects of racism, classism, and other structures of oppression that exist and cause health disparities. We need societal-level programs to create healthy sleep environments for all. Nonetheless, given that this book is meant to empower you with strategies you can start using today, I definitely encourage you to try them out and see if they help. If you suspect that your sleep is poor, don't wait to advocate for yourself with your medical care team.

REFLECT AND SET GOALS: As we bring this chapter to a close, reflect on your sleep quality and its possible role in the chronic pain you're experiencing. What factors present in your life could be making your sleep worse? Which of these are somewhat within your control and modifiable?

Is it possible to incorporate some of the strategies presented in this chapter? List any sleep-related goals that come to mind below or in a journal:

This week: ....

....

This month: ....

....

Over the next six months: ....

....

Supports I need to stick to my goals: ....

....

....

Questions for my doctor: ....

....

....

13

It's Safe to Move

Lowering Inflammation, Pain, and Fear
While Boosting the Reward System

O ne of the most common beliefs I hear among my clients is that moving will trigger a pain episode or harm their body in some way.
Because of this they rest more and move less. This fear is entirely understandable. Your brain sends you pain as a danger warning signal, and
protecting yourself can involve freezing or withdrawing. If your ankle
were throbbing after a sprain, immobilizing yourself might help prevent
further harm. Or retreating indoors might feel safer than going on a hike
or playing softball. But these behaviors make sense only for acute pain.
Chronic pain is much more (if not completely in some cases) about alarm
system hypersensitivity than about tissue damage that needs rest to heal.

Scientific Discoveries about Movement
and Chronic Pain

If you fear movement or believe it isn't right for you when you're experiencing chronic pain, you're not alone, and there are reasons why you
experience these feelings and beliefs. Yet keep in mind this important
principle: *feelings and beliefs are not facts.* This can be tough to remember
when emotions are running high and worrisome thoughts are swirling.
So let's take a look at the facts. Pain scientists have learned a lot about

the relationship between physical activity and chronic pain that counters common beliefs about movement and could free you from fears that are holding you back from greater pain relief.

Physical Activity Has Anti-Inflammatory Effects and Reduces Pain

Physical activity is a broadly defined concept that includes any activity that requires energy expenditure, such as gardening, housework, playing with your kids, swimming, structured exercise, mind–body practices, walking, dancing, and more. It has been shown to reduce inflammation and decrease pain.

Physical Activity Is a Well Behavior

Physical activity can increase your belief that you can do hard things and be persistent. It also may increase your feelings of control over pain and your ability to accept pain rather than go to war with it.

Physical Activity Reduces Fear and Boosts the Reward System

Regular physical activity can reduce anxiety, which you now know tends to ramp up the alarm. It also boosts the reward system, including by increasing the availability of pain-relieving and mood-boosting biochemicals like opioids and serotonin (your body's natural pharmacy!). It promotes positive feelings including self-confidence. Many studies have also shown that regular exercise is an effective treatment for depression, a condition that often shows up alongside chronic pain and is characterized by poor functioning of the reward system.

Physical Inactivity Is Perceived as a Threat by Your Body

The human body is designed to be in regular motion. Some theorists even consider physical movement a basic human need or drive that is akin to sleep and nutrition. So it's not surprising that your body reacts to prolonged inactivity as a threat. As pain neuroscience educators David

Butler and Lorimer Moseley explain, being still for too long leads to a buildup of cellular by-products, including acid, in your tissues. Acid activates the body's danger receptors, which then send a danger message to the brain, thus increasing the chance that the brain will produce pain to motivate you to act (move around). Movement promotes circulation, which delivers oxygen and nutrients to the tissues and clears away acid. Think about how you feel after sitting in the car for a while on a long road trip. Your joints start to feel stiff from inactivity, so you become compelled to pull off the road and stretch your legs at a rest stop, which helps to relieve the pain.

Physical Inactivity Is a Sick-Role Behavior

Sitting or lying down for long periods signals to your brain that you aren't well. A mindset that you're sick and unlikely to get better can start to creep in. If you don't get out into the world and do things, your brain loses the opportunity to learn that you are in fact healthy and safe, capable of doing things you value and that make you feel strong. Physical inactivity is therefore sometimes called a *sick-role behavior* in contrast to *well behaviors*. You want to engage in as many well behaviors as possible, and you want the people in your life to reinforce those well behaviors. Sometimes family or friends inadvertently encourage sick-role behaviors by offering to take over additional household chores and encouraging rest and medication use. These gestures of support are well-intentioned, but support with staying engaged in physical activity best serves chronic pain recovery.

Pacing Activity and Planning Rest Breaks Are Important

A key well behavior in the case of chronic pain is to plan your physical activity so that you, and not your pain level, are in charge of your activity level. It's very common to take rest breaks when you're in pain rather than figuring out in advance when you'll take them. Reacting to pain rather than planning proactively puts pain in control of your behavior. Likewise, activity pacing puts you in charge because you decide ahead of time that you'll take the middle path rather than letting pain dictate that you'll either overdo it or succumb to pain and become sedentary.

One pattern that is *not* the middle path is the boom-bust cycle. This looks like fitting in every errand, chore, and leisure activity you can think of on low- or no-pain days, then crashing into what feels like pain and fatigue disaster afterward.

Another common and unfortunate trajectory is a slow descent into a mostly sedentary lifestyle. As chronic pain persists over months and years, people gradually give up physical activities they loved without modifying them or finding new physical activities that help them maintain muscle mass and cardiovascular fitness despite pain. In this scenario the body becomes deconditioned and far more likely to remain stuck in (or descend further into) a chronic pain state than if physical activity (and therefore muscle mass, cardiovascular fitness, and healthy weight) had been maintained.

As a general guideline, think about how you can break down activities into manageable steps and build in rest breaks between activity bouts. Let's say Ximena enjoys basketball. She knows she can shoot hoops for 15 minutes with a small to moderate increase in pain. She might start by shooting hoops for 10 to 15 minutes at a time, and when the time is up, rest for 10 minutes. She then gradually increases the length of time and number of sessions over a month. Although the process feels frustrating and cumbersome at times and temporary (yet manageable) increases in pain show up at the beginning, at the end of the month she feels satisfied and empowered by how much more she can do and how much less pain and fatigue she experiences.

Movement Breaks or "Snacks" Add Up

Moving in brief bouts throughout the day is an excellent method for increasing activity levels, particularly for those who detest structured exercise. Some research even suggests that moving often throughout the day may support health better than breaking up long periods of sitting with a single intense exercise session. This might look like getting up to move for 5 to 10 minutes every 30 to 60 minutes. If you were to take 10 minutes every hour to, say, walk briskly, do body weight exercises like squats or push-ups, or do housework that involves going up and down stairs over an 8-hour stretch, that equals almost an hour and a half of activity!

You might come across the term *nonexercise activity thermogenesis* or NEAT, which refers to all the energy we expend doing any activity besides resting, eating, and structured exercise. It appears to be very important for our health. Try to think of all the ways you could increase NEAT in your life: playing with your kids outdoors, doing extra household or yard tasks, planting a garden, using a standing desk at work, commuting via bicycle, walking the dog, dancing around your bedroom, and more. If you sit a lot during the day, I recommend setting a timer on your phone (there are apps available for this) to go off every hour, to remind yourself to move. The more you can integrate NEAT into your everyday life, the easier it will be to do consistently. You don't have to do anything special or out of the ordinary to accomplish it.

How to Get Moving: Frequently Asked Questions

You might have a lot of questions about how you can use physical activity to help yourself recover from chronic pain. Here are the most common ones, along with answers from research and clinical experience. The box beginning on the next page provides tips to get you going and keep you going. You might want to make a copy of it and post it somewhere that you'll see often. As always, consult with your care team as you consider new pain management approaches.

Q. What activities are best for pain, and how much should I do?

A. Given that each chronic pain situation is unique, there are no strict guidelines for how, when, and how much physical activity everyone living with chronic pain should do. It appears that a personalized plan tailored to you and your interests, strengths, and limitations is best. In fact, it doesn't take much. Research suggests that even two or three exercise sessions per week over a few weeks can make a real impact on pain as well as mental health, and as discussed earlier, every movement "snack" you do adds to the benefit! Here are some possible activities:

- Strength training: lifting weights, using resistance bands, etc.
- Aerobic exercise: brisk walking or running, swimming, cycling, and the like

- Mind–body exercises: yoga, tai chi, martial arts
- Any sport or other activity that already interests you (hiking?), modified somehow to fit your current abilities
- Intentionally increasing NEAT: playing catch with your kids; doing strenuous housework like mopping, vacuuming, or organizing; taking the stairs instead of the elevator; parking as far away as you can in parking lots; walking or biking to destinations; using a standing desk; taking the dog for an extra walk; doing five quick exercises (squats, jumping jacks, whatever works!) every time you send an email or unload the dishwasher. Be as creative as you can!

Know that the specific type of activity matters less than doing it regularly over the long term. A general consensus among researchers and clinicians appears to be that any movement, no matter how small, is a good thing. Remember that you don't need expensive exercise equipment. Know that walking, if that's available to you, is associated with significant improvements in pain and function.

SCIENCE-BACKED TIPS TO GET YOU GOING

- **Label and challenge inaccurate thoughts that are telling you movement will hurt your body and that being still is the safest bet.** Stick to your physical activity goals in collaboration with your care team.
- **Individually tailor your exercise program to your interests and abilities.** Try to do something you like! Remember that all activities count.
- **Encourage yourself with a positive inner dialogue.** Give yourself credit for every activity you do, even if it's just for five minutes. When you fall short of your physical movement goals, use your self-compassion skills. Self-compassion, not self-criticism, promotes behavior change.
- **Avoid perfectionistic, black-and-white thinking.** If you lie around for three days, avoid thoughts like "I've already let myself go for this long, so what's the point?!" It doesn't need to be perfect—let it be good enough.
- **Challenge beliefs that are no longer serving you.** Sometimes our ideas and beliefs can get in the way of doing physical activity that best supports chronic pain recovery. For instance, Sarah had been a high-achieving professional athlete who grew up learning that failing to achieve perfection in anything (a sport, project, or task) was shameful. When her chronic pain

took root in adulthood, she found herself being held back by these unhelpful, perfectionistic narratives she had learned. She felt that if she couldn't do an extensive weight-training program involving multiple hours of lifting per week, it was no use. However, through therapy, including pain neuroscience education, she came to embrace the idea that every little bit counts, and that increasing activity engagement gradually (as opposed to overdoing it or avoiding it altogether) is a sign of strength (rather than a weakness).

- **Don't wait to "feel" motivated to move.** If you don't "feel" like moving, do it anyway. Remember that we all have unwanted feelings and thoughts that crop up all the time. Don't let these unwanted experiences run the show. Get back in control by focusing instead on taking the actions you want to: you can take the unpleasant "stuff" with you as you engage in physical activity. You might even picture yourself carrying it with you in a backpack—it's there, but it's not in charge. You'll probably find that unwanted thoughts and feelings shift in a more pleasant, positive direction.

- **Keep reasonable expectations for yourself.** Don't expect yourself to make big changes overnight. Remember that transitioning from a sedentary lifestyle to an active one is the hardest part. Once you reach a certain level of fitness, it will become easier to maintain your gains.

- **Move with a group.** When you surround yourself with other people who value physical activity it becomes so much easier to do the same. Look for local walking groups or exercise classes.

- **Remind yourself of risks and rewards.** This is a classic behavior change strategy. We're more likely to engage in healthy behaviors when we think we're at risk of something bad happening and also think something good will happen as a result of our efforts. Remind yourself that sedentary behavior will lead to deconditioning, which makes pain worse and increases the risk of many, many health problems. Remind yourself that physical movement is a science-backed way of turning down pain volume and that temporary activity-induced increases in pain (muscle soreness) are not dangerous.

- **Integrate it into your life.** Think of ways to make it really easy on yourself. Keep some hand weights near the couch. Keep a yoga mat in your office. Promise your dog you'll walk him three times a day. Bike or walk to destinations instead of driving. Consider a standing desk.

- **Use self-monitoring.** As much as we often hate to take a direct look at ourselves, monitoring our behavior is a highly effective way to adopt healthy habits. If it's available to you, try an app or smartwatch that can track your activity (like daily steps).

- **Believe in yourself as best you can.** You can do it!

Q. Is it safe?

A. Yes. It is widely documented that exercise and physical activity interventions are safe for people living with chronic pain.

Q. I'm ready to get more active. What does the process look like?

A. Experts recommend a gradual approach to increasing activity levels that keeps activity pacing and planned rest breaks in mind. Ideally, you would engage in this process under the supervision of a qualified professional like a physical therapist or physiotherapist, since having an expert to coach and guide you through the process has been shown to help people stick with their plan and succeed.

Say you want to be able to mow your own lawn. Instead of suddenly trying to mow the entire lawn on a given day after not having done it for about a year, make a plan that helps you pace the activity. This could look like mowing for 20 minutes a day over the course of three days and lying down to practice 10 minutes of mindful meditation or slow breathing after your 20 minutes of mowing. Doing something like this might feel frustrating because it's so far from how you used to be; before you had a chronic pain condition, you could just get up and go. Bring compassion to any feelings of frustration, hopelessness, or loss as you consider new ways of increasing activity levels that will work in your current circumstances and set you on a path to feeling better.

Q. I'm sad that I can't do everything that I used to be able to do without thinking. How can I deal with this?

A. It can be hard to accept that you might not be able to do the same activities you used to or to the same degree. I felt like I had to give up certain forms of strenuous exercise for a while because they were so overwhelming to my sensory system. The bright lights at the gym, loud music, and 5:00 a.m. workouts simply weren't in the cards when my pain was at its worst. I found that yoga and swimming were still enjoyable and relieved my pain a bit, so I did those activities often. James really struggled to set goals around activity pacing, because doing so reminded him of how much he'd lost to his chronic pain condition. He was once an elite baseball player, and the ability to be strong and capable in most situations had been a big part of his identity. Naming the grief was important. He then looked for creative ways to help himself get going. He decided to involve his spouse in his goal-setting process. They started a tree-planting project together, which turned out to be a way of kick-starting a new, more flexible physical activity plan. In general, you can allow yourself to grieve what you wish you could do at a given time and seek new activities that work. Be proud of every effort you make and be compassionate and kind to yourself.

Q. Does it matter if my pain is mild, moderate, or severe?

A. No. Physical activity can benefit people living with severe pain as well as mild and moderate pain.

Q. Shouldn't I rest during flares?

A. Experts generally recommend continuing to find ways to avoid completely sedentary behavior (such as staying in bed all day) when you experience a pain flare. For instance, maybe you don't do an exercise session at the gym but still take the dog for a 15-minute walk. Although becoming completely inactive may be tempting when pain flares up, doing so repeatedly can easily rob you of strength and aerobic capacity, as well as create more physical limitations.

Q. What if my pain goes up after I exercise?

A. Remember that increased muscle soreness is normal after doing physical activities that you aren't in the habit of doing. Some experts offer the general guideline that muscle soreness—soreness in the belly of the muscle 24 hours after exercise—is acceptable even if it's uncomfortable. However, pain in a tendon, ligament, or joint is not OK, and a major pain flare with exercise is not OK either. It can be hard to tell whether the pain you're feeling after activity reflects muscle soreness or something else; here it becomes critical to consult with a physical therapist or other qualified professional for personalized guidance. A professional can help you avoid the extremes of overdoing or avoiding activity as you work to build up your physical activity and fitness levels. Use your self-compassion skills every step of the way.

Q. What if I feel anxious as I try to move more?

A. Once you have some guidance and a plan in place, try not to let fear hold you back. Jenny was a tennis player who was struggling with chronic back pain. Although she had been cleared to compete by her physical therapist and athletic trainer, she still found herself playing scared, afraid of damaging her body in some way. She wasn't having fun, and she was playing some pretty bad tennis. She was struggling to trust her trainer's assessment that in her case, *hurt* (familiar chronic pain sensations) while playing did not mean *harm* (new tissue damage). She and I talked about pain neuroscience and the faulty alarm system concept. It seemed that her alarm system (pain-related worry) had gotten stuck in high gear. She started saying to herself, *Thanks brain, for trying to keep me safe. But I'm OK. It's safe to hit the ball hard and go for it.* She also used mindfulness to help herself stay present: she practiced labeling worry-based thoughts as movie plots, rather than reality. She worked hard to focus her mind on her game, rather than her pain. She stayed in close contact with the athletic training staff and followed their recommendations. Over a couple of months she started to see major increases in her confidence, performance, and enjoyment of the sport. You may or may not identify as an athlete, but Jenny's story shows how challenging fear-based thoughts and using mindfulness techniques can help you stay in the game (your physical activity plan) when anxiety shows up.

Q. What if I really can't get myself to get up and go?

A. When your pain is flaring it might feel like nothing will help. Emily would often get stuck in feelings of helplessness and in catastrophic thinking patterns when her back pain would flare. *I'll probably miss work tomorrow. I thought the medications were working, but here we go again. I might lose my job soon.* All she would want to do would be to curl up in a dark room and sob. One thing that helped her was to identify and do the "bare minimum" to stop participating in the vicious cycle of increased pain, rumination, and stopping activity. It often felt forced, but she would do something small like take out the trash or do Pilates for five minutes. Over time, she began to feel like these kinds of "bare minimums" were adding up, and she started to feel more empowered and in control. When you feel like you can't do a thing, do the bare minimum.

ENVIRONMENTAL IRRITANTS

Now that you've learned about the importance of nutrition, sleep, and physical activity, consider the role of the environment in which you live. Every chronic pain condition is embedded within the environment: our health, or lack thereof, doesn't exist in a vacuum. Our living conditions expose us to pollutants (indoor and outdoor), ultra-processed foods with few nutrients, abundant opportunities to consume inflammatory substances (such as nicotine and large amounts of alcohol), endless opportunities to sit around indoors, and various chemicals with potentially harmful effects (think the unpronounceable ingredients found in cleaning products, fertilizers, pesticides, cosmetics, artificial fragrances, plastics, and the like).

Our bodies aren't prepared to handle these sorts of conditions. In fact, there is a mismatch between our genes and our present-day environment. Genetically, the body is designed for life in the Paleolithic Era (beginning about two and a half million years ago), which was characterized by clean air; exposure to diverse microorganisms via plants, soil, and animals (important for a healthy microbiome); an active lifestyle that included walking, lifting, and climbing; and a healthy diet consisting of meat, fruit, and vegetables. Unfortunately, the climate and plastics crises are only increasing the likelihood that our bodies will encounter insults we weren't designed to handle, with real health consequences as a result. Why are chronic pain conditions on the rise? Arguably, our changing environmental circumstances may play a role. There are things we can all do, however, to live in a cleaner environment (see the box on the next page).

Of course, we need policy-level change to create a healthier environment for all. But along with a healthier diet, better sleep, and increased physical activity, the steps in the following box may support your health.

THINGS WE CAN ALL DO
TO LIVE IN A CLEANER ENVIRONMENT

Although we would need to cease existing to avoid all environmental health risk factors, here are some suggested strategies to support a cleaner environment for yourself and your family (and our planet):

- **Clean up your everyday household products.** Find cleaning and other products that are safer for you, your family members, and the planet by looking for the "Safer Choice" label, which is regulated by the U.S. Environmental Protection Agency. Choose unscented products when possible. You can make an inexpensive, safer cleaning solution for your home by simply mixing equal parts vinegar and water in a spray bottle. Also, castile soap and water go a long way. If you make a homemade cleaning solution, be sure to label it!

- **Refrain from using nicotine and reduce your alcohol consumption.** These substances increase your risk of experiencing pain, fatigue, and noncommunicable diseases such as cancer.

- **Reduce exposure to plastics.** Look for ways to cut plastic out of your life. It's basically everywhere, so this is a tough one. Opt for reusable bags and containers. Try to buy foods at markets or stores that aren't wrapped in plastic. Consider plastic-free storage containers. If you need to buy new clothes, opt for plastic-free and environmentally friendlier fabrics such as TENCEL (Lyocell) or linen.

- **Use a high-quality water filter.** Filtering your water can help remove contaminants.

- **Eat organic if your budget allows.** Research suggests that organic foods have lower levels of synthetic fertilizer, pesticide residues, and heavy metals that can be detrimental to our health. Fight climate change and get physically active by growing some of your own food.

- **Do what you can about air pollution.** Open your windows if you can each day to let some fresh air in and get outside as much as possible. Consider an indoor air purifier and grow indoor plants to promote better indoor air quality. Contribute to efforts to improve outdoor air pollution by biking, walking, using public transit, or opting for an electric vehicle.

PART FIVE

WIDENING THE LENS
Building a Holistic Pain Self-Management Plan

M any people live with chronic pain for years, believing that pills and procedures are the only means to recover from it. If you've made it this far, you know how far that is from the truth. You now appreciate how important it is to retrain the brain, adopt new behaviors, address your social well-being, and chip away at the problem with persistence. You need to view your recovery process not like a straight line, nor as an ongoing search for the one magic bullet that will make it better. Pain is a complex, biopsychosocial problem that requires multiple healing strategies. You already have many important tools in your toolbox. In Chapter 14 you'll expand your knowledge even further by learning about integrative pain care, which is the recommended approach for chronic pain management. You'll learn about complementary health-care approaches that have helped others and learn communication tools that can help you collaborate with your care team and with health insurers. In Chapter 15 you'll move forward with a plan. You will integrate *all* your new knowledge and skills and organize them into daily, weekly, monthly and yearly goals. You will design your own unique, upward spiral toward pain relief and greater well-being. Reading about the strategies is not enough; they need to become habits. You can do it!

14

Integrative Pain Care

The experience of chronic pain is impacted by so many complex factors that one treatment isn't likely to be sufficient. Therefore, pain experts recommend an integrative approach to pain management. *Integrative* means combining two or more treatments in a manner that is coordinated, collaborative, interdisciplinary, and personalized. In other words, different providers work together to optimize treatment for each individual patient.

Integrative care also often involves combining *complementary* treatments with conventional Western medical treatments in a coordinated way. Complementary treatments are evidence-based health-care approaches that have been historically considered outside the "mainstream" Western medical paradigm. Think of them as additional tools that may help calm a sensitive pain alarm. Combining chiropractic care, psychotherapy, nutrition therapy, and pharmaceuticals (medication) is one basic example of what integrative pain care can look like.

Research suggests that complementary treatments can favorably impact your nervous system, including inflammatory processes and the brain. An integrative approach to pain management is aligned with the recommendations of research and health-care authorities including the National Institute of Health's National Pain Strategy and the Department of Health and Human Services Pain Management Best Practices. Research suggests that treatment approaches like chiropractic care, manual therapy, yoga and tai chi, acupuncture, functional medicine, neuromodulation (the alteration of nervous system activity by way of electrical currents, magnetic pulses, or chemicals), photobiomodulation (light therapies), and others can make a real impact. So, in collaboration with your care team, you may be interested in pursuing an integrative plan.

The challenge: studies show that Americans' use of complementary health-care approaches is on the rise, and pain management is an oft-cited reason for use. But you should be aware that insurance companies still (as of this writing) tend to pay more for medications than complementary approaches like manual therapy or acupuncture. Many have called for payors to reimburse integrative pain management programs that include complementary medicine. Although it's an uphill battle, the demand for complementary treatments appears to be rising, and research shows that the amount Americans are spending on complementary treatments has increased significantly in recent years. Increased demand might prompt more insurance plans to cover complementary care. And complementary approaches offer an effective alternative to opioid therapy, which has its risks (although it can be a lifesaver for some—as always, pain treatment should be personalized). As the United States battles an opioid crisis, opioid-free therapies, including complementary approaches, have an increasing appeal among several stakeholders.

It can be difficult in our health-care system to get providers to talk to one another and coordinate care. In my experience the task of piecing together an integrative pain management program often falls on the person living with pain. This means that you need to actively tell all your providers which treatments you're using and suggest new treatments that you might like to try. Ask if they have guidance on how to use them in an integrated way. Don't wait for the doctor to ask you specific questions about your overall treatment plan: volunteer as much information and ask as many questions as you can. If possible take someone else with you to your appointments who can help advocate for you.

On the following pages you'll read about some of the more common evidence-based complementary approaches so you can get an idea of what is currently out there. Later in the chapter I offer some tips on how to increase affordability and communicate effectively with your providers. Expect to encounter some barriers to getting the treatments you want to try but be persistent and trust that your efforts to build an integrative care plan for yourself will likely benefit you.

Complementary Treatment Approaches: The Big Picture

This chapter does not offer medical advice but rather provides educational information for your consideration in collaboration with your care team. Here is some "big picture" information about complementary approaches that are generally considered safe and effective. After each treatment I include practical tips related to costs and insurance.

Manual Therapies

Manual therapy consists of treatments in which a trained clinician (chiropractor, massage therapist, physical therapist, osteopath, athletic trainer, occupational therapist) uses their hands or instruments to apply a physical stimulus to the body. Clinical pain care guidelines recognize manual therapy as an evidence-based treatment that can be used in conjunction with other types of treatment. Massage therapy and spinal manipulation (often a part of chiropractic care) are two widely practiced manual therapies that can favorably impact pain and daily functioning:

- Massage involves hands-on manipulation of the body's soft tissue and may help with neck and shoulder pain, some fibromyalgia symptoms, and knee osteoarthritis, although the effects may be short term.
- Spinal manipulation involves delivering a controlled thrust to a joint in the spine, the force of which moves the joint more than it would without it. Spinal manipulation is most commonly performed by chiropractors, but physical therapists and osteopathic physicians can also offer it. It can be helpful for low back pain, neck pain, headache, and sciatica, and serious side effects are rare.

Why exactly manual therapies can be helpful for chronic pain is still under investigation. Current theories point to the idea that they produce physiological responses (including brain responses and changes in inflammation) that ultimately alter the experience of pain. Furthermore, the providers are often adept at conveying warmth and empathy, which can be healing in its own right.

Costs, Insurance, and Practical Tips

- Among complementary treatments, chiropractic care is the most frequently covered by insurance.
- Some insurance plans cover massage if it's deemed medically necessary by a doctor (see the box on pages 150–151).
- Physical therapy is often covered by insurance, and many physical therapists incorporate massage and spinal manipulation into a treatment regimen. When shopping around for physical therapy practices, ask if they incorporate massage techniques and spinal manipulation.

Meditative Movement Practices

Several meditative practices integrate mind–body awareness, breathing practices, and movement. Discussed below are two of the most commonly studied:

- Tai chi is an ancient martial art that originated in China and has been adopted in the United States to support health and physical rehabilitation. It involves slow and gentle movements, controlled breathing, and the cultivation of a meditative state of mind. A small amount of research suggests that regular practice of tai chi can help osteoarthritis, lower back pain, and fibromyalgia symptoms.

- Yoga is an ancient spiritual practice originating in India, and elements of it have become popular in the United States to improve physical and mental health. There is a vast array of yoga styles, ranging from the gentle to the more physically rigorous. A small number of studies suggest that yoga is a promising practice for pain, including neck pain, headaches, and knee osteoarthritis. It may also help pain indirectly via reducing stress and increasing well-being.

Meditative movement practices can reduce inflammation, which could be because of how they can reduce stress via the combination of meditation, relaxation, and movement. If you're drawn to these practices, they can be a great way of incorporating both movement and meditation into a weekly routine.

Costs, Insurance, and Practical Tips

- Yoga and tai chi usually aren't covered by insurance. But these activities are generally affordable if you take group classes, and they're often offered as part of a gym membership. You can also search for free videos online. Once you learn the techniques, you can do them on your own at any time for free. As always, consult your care team before starting a new pain care approach.

Neuromodulation Therapies

As we've explored throughout the book, you can change your brain by practicing new mental habits and behaviors. Neuromodulation (altering nerve activity through targeted delivery of stimuli) is another way of changing how the brain works, this one involving applying inputs like electrical currents and magnetic pulses. Various neuromodulation techniques are available; the more invasive techniques involve implanting a device within the body and less invasive approaches use a device that is located outside the body. Spinal cord stimulation is one of the more common neuromodulation therapies for pain and involves surgically implanting a device that sends a mild electrical current into the spinal cord to relieve pain. It is generally used for severe pain that hasn't responded to other therapies. Transcranial magnetic stimulation, or TMS, is a generally safe and noninvasive way of sending magnetic pulses into the brain to change how it processes pain. It does not require surgery. The TMS device, located outside the body, produces brief magnetic pulses that pass through the skull and into the cortex, or the outer layer of the brain. TMS has been shown to help with several pain conditions, including migraine, fibromyalgia, nociplastic pain, and others.

Costs, Insurance, and Practical Tips

- If your doctor deems TMS medically necessary you may be able to get some insurance coverage. Ask your insurance carrier using the prompts listed at the end of the chapter. If you can't get any coverage, TMS is usually prohibitively expensive.

- The FDA has approved TMS for depression. People living with chronic pain often also meet criteria for depression at some point during their pain journey. If you have a depression diagnosis your insurance might cover TMS to treat it. The insurance company might require that you try other depression treatments first (such as oral medications). Treating depression through TMS or other approaches has the potential to help chronic pain.

- The FDA has approved an at-home TMS device, often referred to as single pulse transcranial magnetic stimulation (sTMS), for migraine. Taking insurance out of the equation, it's way cheaper than provider-administered TMS. At the time of this writing, companies selling the device market it at around $400 per month. If you ever speak to a drug or device manufacturer about their products, ask if they have any discount programs.

- Spinal cord stimulation is often covered by major insurers.

Acupuncture

Acupuncture was developed within the ancient practice of traditional Chinese medicine, which was developed over thousands of years to prevent and treat disease and is now used worldwide. Acupuncture involves placing hair-thin needles into the skin at specified points along the body, which are then activated by the provider's hands or through electrical stimulation. Acupuncture can impact the nervous system (including the brain and brain biochemicals that can alter pain and positive emotions, including internal opioids; it might also help reduce inflammation). Needle stimulation can impact brain activity not only in areas that process sensations of touch but also in areas involved in our emotions and thinking patterns. Given that chronic pain impacts and is impacted by our thoughts and emotions, these findings are interesting and promising. Overall, research suggests that acupuncture is generally safe and effective for several pain conditions when performed by a qualified provider. As with manual therapies, rich healing ritual is often involved in acupuncture treatment, as well as positive and collaborative provider–patient interactions (think safety signals to the brain).

Costs, Insurance, and Practical Tips

- By some estimates around 30 percent of major insurers cover acupuncture, so it's worth calling yours to find out what they cover.

- Acupuncturists increasingly offer "community acupuncture," where they treat several patients at once in a large room. It really drives the cost down. Search online for "community acupuncture" in your area.

- Do an internet search for local acupuncture schools and see if they offer discounted rates to work with an advanced student under the supervision of a licensed provider.

Photobiomodulation

Can we use light to heal our bodies and minds? Based on numerous scientific studies over the past decade, the answer appears to be yes. Photobiomodulation refers to altering biological processes (including brain processes) using light. Light, in its various forms, supports our emotional and biological functioning in crucial ways. For example, light and darkness impact our circadian rhythm and the production of biochemicals like serotonin and melatonin, which impact our mood, sleep, and alertness. Sunlight exposure prompts the body to produce vitamin D (low vitamin D levels have been linked to poorer health outcomes, with some research hinting at links between vitamin D and chronic pain). Meanwhile, changes in our relationship with light over the course of our human history have created health risks. We manufacture all sorts of artificial light and shine it on ourselves to excess: we spend hours upon hours a day staring at screens (blue light), which disrupts circadian rhythm, while our exposure to light at night has simply increased due to street and city lights. Our routines can be completely divorced from the rising and setting sun, and we thus aren't exposed to red light (think sunrise and sunset) the way our ancestors were.

Light is received and processed biologically not just through the eyes but also through the skin. Researchers have examined the pain-relieving and pain-exacerbating effects of light of different wavelengths (white, red, near infrared, green, and blue) delivered visually and to the skin (shone on a small, painful area of the body like the jaw, or over the entire body). Overall, light therapies may help with several pain conditions including fibromyalgia, complex regional pain syndrome, temporomandibular disorder, and chronic low back pain. Photobiomodulation is considered a safe and noninvasive treatment with favorable effects on inflammation, oxidative stress, tissue healing, circulation, and brain biochemicals including serotonin. Green light therapy might be particularly promising for fibromyalgia, while red and near infrared light therapy may have anti-inflammatory and fatigue-reducing effects.

If you're interested in trying out photobiomodulation, consult your health-care team. Moreover, be sure to support your healing potential with light naturally. As recommended earlier in the book, go outside every day and intentionally enjoy the peaceful green sights. Minimize your contact with screens (blue light) as much as possible, particularly late in the day, and sleep in a dark room without artificial light shining in (consider blackout curtains or an eye mask). Stay tuned for more research on this fascinating way of supporting our health!

Costs, Insurance, and Practical Tips

- Whole-body red or infrared light therapy devices are a one-time purchase (usually a few hundred dollars; see for example *https://orionrlt. com*), and you can self-administer the treatment at home. You can use the device for as long as it continues to work. This is much cheaper than relying on provider visits for treatments. Before purchasing a device, consult your health-care team.

- Insurance does not generally cover photobiomodulation therapy for pain, despite its established clinical evidence.

Functional Medicine

Functional medicine is a model of health care that uses a "root cause" approach to identify and treat things that trigger illnesses, including imbalances in the microbiome, allergens, infections, stress, genetic factors, and poor diet, while helping people optimize health-supportive lifestyle factors like diet, relationships, physical activity, and sleep. Functional medicine incorporates multiple evidence-based strategies that target biopsychosocial factors in a deep, coordinated, and personalized way. Nutrition therapy is considered a first-line treatment.

Functional medicine is not in opposition to conventional medicine but rather a partner to it. Functional medicine providers have a license in a conventional medical discipline (medical doctor, physician assistant, registered nurse) and also receive advanced training in assessing and treating root causes of illnesses like microbiome-related factors. Functional medicine providers take a comprehensive medical history and lifestyle assessment and collaborate with patients to establish a personalized, integrative, and holistic treatment plan. Emerging research indicates that functional medicine can support better health and quality of life. Notably, the Cleveland Clinic established a dedicated functional medicine clinic in their academic medical center in 2014, the Center for Functional Medicine (*https://my.clevelandclinic.org/departments/functional-medicine*). The center offers virtual appointments, as well as an innovative 10-week group program with condition-specific tracks, such as autoimmune conditions and digestive disorders. More commonly, functional medicine providers work in private practice. Find a provider certified in functional medicine at The Institute for Functional Medicine's website, *www.ifm.org/find-a-practitioner*. I personally believe that the functional medicine model is the future of health care, particularly when it comes to treating (and even reversing) chronic illness.

Costs, Insurance, and Practical Tips

- Be prepared to try to use your out-of-network benefits (if you have them) for functional medicine, but it's possible that some functional medicine providers will be in-network with insurers. If you locate a functional medicine provider you'd like to get to know more, I recommend asking if they provide a receipt to submit to insurance companies. Then call your insurance company and ask if that specific provider's services would be reimbursed at all by the company.

- Check out the Cleveland Clinic's group appointments model mentioned on the previous page.

Dosing Yourself with the Placebo Effect

Pain researchers continue to investigate the placebo effect, for good reason. Placebo effects, also termed *nonspecific treatment effects* (driven by factors such as medical rituals, strong patient–provider bonds, and expectations) are not "sham" effects—they're legitimate. They can have "real" effects on the experience of pain and even on biological processes that contribute to the pain experience (such as the functioning of our body's natural painkillers). Every treatment, ranging from the most conventional to the most alternative, can work for someone because of specific qualities of that treatment. For example, an anti-inflammatory drug reduces bodily inflammation and therefore pain. Some nonspecific ingredients inherent in a variety of treatments also help. There's the ritual of taking a pill, the positive and culturally embedded expectations we hold around that ritual and being followed by an attentive physician. Placebo effects aren't going to cure brain tumors, but they can have a substantial effect on subjective symptoms like pain and mood.

Interestingly, you might find placebo or nonspecific treatment components far more "potent" in the context of complementary medical care than in a conventional doctor's office. Practitioners of complementary therapies tend to create supportive, calming environments along with positive patient–provider relationships that cue the brain that you're in a healing environment. These cues might help the brain alter its predictions. For instance, bodily sensations might be interpreted as innocuous as opposed to threatening. If you consider adding complementary therapies to your treatment plan, have confidence in the fact that the placebo or nonspecific treatment effects are powerful forces in addition to whatever treatment-specific benefits you may reap.

How to Collaborate with Your Care Providers to Arrive at an Integrated Plan

Here are some tips and strategies for arriving at a collaborative integrated plan:

- Always communicate with your care team before pursuing any new approach and make sure to tell everyone involved in your care which treatments you're using.
- If you want to try a new treatment, ask your doctor about what they see as the pros and cons and advocate for yourself (see Step 2 in the box on page 151).
- Be diligent in evaluating any new provider's qualifications and experience.
- Remember that each chronic pain situation is unique and that it takes some trial and error to figure out what works for you.
- Try your best to get your insurance to pay for some or all of the treatment of interest. You'll find a step-by-step overview in the box on pages 150–151.
- Keep detailed records of your medications, treatments you're using, and treatments you'd like to learn more about. A worksheet for this purpose appears at the back of the book on pages 165–168.
- Sometimes companies that are marketing a device or medication offer coupons or financial assistance. Call the manufacturer directly to ask about this.
- Without dealing with your insurance at all, try to look for discounts directly from providers.
    - If you call a complementary care provider's office, ask "Do you offer any sliding scale pricing, discounts, or coupons?"
    - Look for treatments offered in a group setting.
    - Google graduate training clinics in your area (acupuncture, massage) to see if they offer discounted services from advanced trainees under supervision by licensed professionals. This can often be very affordable.

- Out-of-network benefits can really help.
  - Don't assume that a provider's being out of network means you can't get reimbursed. Many insurance companies will reimburse a large portion (60–70%) of services from out-of-network providers after you meet your out-of-network deductible.
- Establish a budget for your chronic pain care and look in detail at costs and benefits. How much are you currently spending per year on co-pays, facility fees, and bills you didn't expect, and how beneficial are those treatments? Consider this question as you think about your budget and overall treatment goals. Remember, just because something isn't covered by your insurance doesn't mean it will be more expensive than something that is. For example, the out-of-pocket costs you would incur with an invasive conventional treatment might end up being more than three months of regular massage therapy.

SEEKING INSURANCE REIMBURSEMENT FOR COMPLEMENTARY CARE

- Step 1. Learn about your benefits
  - Call the number on the back of your insurance card to talk to customer service. Ask "Is there any coverage for _____ treatment under my insurance plan if my physician says it's medically necessary?"
    - If the answer is yes, ask:
      - "What providers are covered to administer the treatment? Does the provider need to be in-network? What credentials does the provider need to have? Where can I find a list of in-network providers?"
      - "If I use an out-of-network provider, what percentage of the treatment will be covered? How do I submit a claim after receiving a treatment, and what information needs to be on the receipt from the provider?"
    - "How do I provide documentation of medical necessity to you? Do I upload the letter from my doctor to the patient portal, or can I fax it?"
  - If the insurance company states that they might cover any portion of the treatment so long as you have a letter of medical necessity and/or

a prescription from a physician, have a conversation with your doctor (see Step 2).

- Step 2. Talk with your doctor
  - Explain your interest in a particular treatment. For example: "I recently read in a chronic pain self-help book that _____ treatment can help chronic pain. What do you think the pros and cons of _____ treatment might be in my case?"
  - If they think the treatment may be worth a try, state: "It sounds like there's some uncertainty, but that it might help me. Therefore, I'd like to work with a licensed provider that offers _____ treatment to see if it may help. Would you recommend this for me?"
  - If they agree, ask: "Can you write me a letter of medical necessity for this treatment? I will need to give this to my insurance company. Also, can you write me a prescription or referral for the treatment?"
  - Ask: "Do you recommend any clinics or providers that offer the treatment?"
    - Once you have these documents, give them to your insurance company.
- Step 3. Talk with complementary care providers
  - Ask: "What are your qualifications and credentials? Are you licensed to practice in my state?"
  - Ask: "Are you in-network with my insurance provider, and do you bill them directly on my behalf?"
  - If they aren't in-network, state: "Can you provide me a detailed superbill that I can use to seek reimbursement from insurance?" *Note: A superbill is more than a basic receipt showing that you paid a health-care provider. It is a document that gives you the detailed information you need about the health-care services you pay out-of-pocket for, so that your insurance company can reimburse you. You will use the superbill to submit a claim. The superbill should contain: (1) your (the patient's) information, (2) provider's information, (3) dates of service, (4) procedure codes (CPT codes), (5) diagnosis codes (ICD-10 codes), and (6) fees paid by you to the provider. To avoid delays later on, try to make sure your superbill has these elements before submitting a claim.*
  - Ask: "Insurance aside, do you offer any discounts, sliding scale pricing, or group interventions that might be more affordable?"

Curious about Psychedelics and Medical Cannabis?

Psychedelics and medical cannabis for chronic pain and mental health are receiving a great deal of public and media interest. Here is some big-picture information about what we know and don't know.

Psychedelics

The use of what Western medicine has termed *psychedelic* ("mind-manifesting") substances to alleviate human suffering originates in Indigenous healing traditions around the world (sometimes referred to in the English language as Spirit, traditional, or sacred medicines). In the Western medical context, psychedelics such as psilocybin (the active ingredient in "magic mushrooms"), MDMA ("ecstasy"), and LSD are under investigation for their potential pain-relieving effects. Research suggests that they can favorably impact mental health conditions that often happen alongside chronic pain (anxiety, depression, and PTSD). Psychedelic substances often promote experiences of nondual aware-ness or oneness, mystical experiences, or the arising of other personally meaningful insights, which can promote psychospiritual development, enhanced well-being, and improved mental health. Data from a hand-ful of studies suggest that using psychedelic substances in a therapeutic context (such as with a trained guide or therapist) may produce large, durable, and rapid reductions in depression, reduce existential fear of death in people with life-threatening illness, and improve symptoms of other psychiatric disorders. Research continues to investigate the degree to which psychedelics may outperform traditional Western medical treat-ments for mental health conditions.

Research on psychedelics for pain is in its beginning stages. Case studies and small trials indicate possible benefits, and randomized clini-cal trials (rigorous studies that compare a psychedelic substance to a placebo treatment) are currently underway and necessary to investigate the risks and benefits of psychedelics for chronic pain management. At this point we know very little about whether psychedelics may be a good treatment option for chronic pain. Some researchers have theorized that psychedelics could improve pain via neurobiological, psychospiritual, or anti-inflammatory mechanisms, but again, more research is needed. You may have heard the term *microdosing*. This refers to taking small amounts of psychedelic substances such that a mystical or hallucinatory experience does not emerge. Whether a mystical experience is required to benefit from psychedelics (or if a very small dose is beneficial) remains to be seen.

Leading experts on psychedelic science have cautioned that psychedelics research currently finds itself in a moment of overinflated expectations regarding the health benefits of psychedelics driven by media and industry (some forecast the investment potential of psychedelic medicines reaching billions of dollars). As you're probably aware, psychedelic medicine in the United States has fallen in and out of favor over the past century in reaction to political, social, and media influences and has been subjected to extreme views (miracle or madness). Our current moment of overinflated expectations may be followed by a period of cultural disillusionment with psychedelic medicines and ultimately (hopefully) by a middle path of realistic expectations and productive use of these medicines backed by science.

Perhaps most important, to the detriment of psychedelic science research, Indigenous voices and leadership have been largely absent from Western psychedelics research, and there is a general lack of recognition of the sacred cultural positioning of these medicines, cultural appropriation, and patenting of traditional medicines for profit. Embracing diverse knowledge systems as we continue to learn more about the therapeutic effects of psychedelics in medical treatment settings will ensure the greatest benefit for all communities involved. There is an urgent need for Western scientists to work ethically and respectfully with Indigenous leaders and cultures from whence the recognition of the benefit of these plants, combined with the spiritual practices and rituals surrounding their use, originated. Psychedelics are promising for pain, yet systematic research that is culturally sensitive, inclusive, ethical, and embracing of Indigenous wisdom will serve best.

If you're interested in psychedelics for pain, consult your medical care team and stay tuned for more science-backed information and recommendations. Treating any health condition with psychedelics requires doing so safely under the guidance of an ongoing clinical trial or medical care team.

Medical Cannabis

Cannabis refers to all products originating from the cannabis plant. According to the National Institutes of Health, cannabis contains hundreds of different chemical substances. Cannabinoids are one group of substances found in cannabis, and the most well-known cannabinoids are THC (Delta-9-tetrahydrocannabinol) and CBD (cannabidiol). Other cannabinoids (CBG, CBN) have recently gained popular media attention and are marketed in cannabis products, but very little is known about them. Synthetic cannabinoids (not originating in a plant) also exist. Cannabinoids bind with receptors in our body's own internal endocannabinoid system (which also produces its own natural cannabinoids). The endocannabinoid system plays a role in a vast array of biological and socioemotional processes, including but not limited to mood, pain, how we bond with others, our thinking patterns, and our immune system function (including inflammation). Scientists have long been interested in the question of whether cannabis products can be used therapeutically to address pain, mood disorders, and other conditions.

The numerous ways in which cannabis products are prepared, from their route of administration (smoked, topical, edible, vaporized) to the various concentrations of cannabinoids (THC versus CBD), render them very difficult to study in the classic randomized controlled trial, which likes to isolate a single pharmacological agent and observe its effects relative to placebo treatment. Some studies have, however, begun to investigate medications with only THC or only CBD as the active ingredient (dronabinol, Epidiolex) for pain. These studies might pave the way for future studies on smoking cannabis for medical reasons and similar products that can be bought in a medical cannabis dispensary. Neither of the medications mentioned above have FDA approval to treat pain.

Overall, whether cannabis exerts favorable medical effects and for whom is an extraordinarily complex question. The collection of randomized controlled trials to date on cannabis doesn't offer a clear conclusion on whether it helps pain, with some suggesting a small benefit and others reporting no effect. Contrary to popular belief, cannabis carries a risk of dependence, and side effects also pose a challenge. That said, as you're probably aware, a lot of people with chronic pain use cannabis to manage their symptoms and feel that it helps them. More rigorous research is needed into if, how, and for whom medical cannabis may be helpful. If you're interested in trying medical cannabis for pain, consult your medical care team and stay tuned for more science-backed information and recommendations.

Costs, Insurance, and Practical Tips

- Insurance companies do not typically cover medical cannabis.

- The process to obtain a medical cannabis prescription varies by state. Do an internet search (type "medical cannabis" and the name of your state) for an official website authored by your state's government (often appended with *.gov*) to find out more about the necessary steps in your state. You can also ask other members of your pain care team, as they may have knowledge or experience from having worked with other patients in your area.

How Do I Choose Which Complementary Treatments to Pursue?

Given that each chronic pain case is unique, we don't have a general road map for which treatment to add and when. Your medical care team should help you figure out what's causing your pain and, using that understanding of *your* pain mechanisms, help you decide which additional treatments might be worth a shot. Your best bet is to educate yourself about options that are out there that have an accumulated or emerging evidence base and ask your care team what they think about the risks and benefits in your unique case. Of course, consider also the costs (time, transportation, financial) and how interested in or motivated you feel to pursue the treatment.

In closing, think of each new approach you add as an incremental step toward healing. If a new treatment or strategy reduces your pain by a small percentage, that can still be a win. That bit of pain relief might make it feel more feasible to adopt additional healing strategies, setting an upward spiral in motion. For instance, if chiropractic care reduces your pain by 5 or 10 percent, you might feel a bit more like doing physical activity, which in turn lowers your pain, and so on and so forth.

**FOR FURTHER INFORMATION
ON INTEGRATIVE PAIN CARE**

This chapter has presented some big-picture information about integrative pain care based on current scientific literature and summary statements provided by the National Institute for Complementary and Integrative Health and the International Association for the Study of Pain. Statements made by these organizations are highly reputable, and you can consider them trusted sources for up-to-date information. There are many more complementary and emerging pain treatments that might be useful "ingredients" in an integrative pain care plan than could be reviewed in a single chapter. To read about a vast array of pain treatments with bite-sized explanations, and to create a printable list of treatments that spark your interest to discuss further with your care team, look up "MyPainPlan" on the U.S. Pain Foundation's website (*https://mypainplan.org/mypainplan*). It is an interactive website where you can learn about 85-plus treatments across five categories. Consult the Resources at the end of this book for additional guidance on where to look for trusted information about integrative pain care. A blank form you can fill in for your health-care providers is at the back of the book on pages 165–168 and also available to download at *www.guilford.com/hunt-forms*.

15

Going Forward—with a Plan

I f you've read everything in the book to this point, you've encountered a lot of new information.

I hope you've found a lot of options for lowering your pain alarm volume by retraining your brain and building new habits and strategies that nurture your body and mind. In closing I invite you to reflect on your experience with reading this book and brainstorm a holistic plan for yourself. A holistic pain self-management plan involves building new mental and behavioral habits as well as practicing letting go of things that are no longer serving you.

Creating Your Holistic Pain Self-Management Plan

To recap: first you were introduced to pain neuroscience (pain as an alarm system), threats that can ramp up pain alarms, and sources of joy and meaning that can quiet pain alarms.

What important new understandings of chronic pain have you taken from this book? Jot them down here or in a journal if you like.

....

....

Next, several different pain management approaches that follow directly from a modern scientific understanding of chronic pain were described. Science robustly shows that mental habits, behavior patterns, emotions, and social dynamics can lower pain alarm system hypersensitivity. We reviewed ways of retraining your brain, changing your behavior, and addressing your social well-being for the purpose of lowering pain—treatment based on the biopsychosocial model of pain. Here are some highlights:

- Mindfulness and meditation
- Identifying thoughts, beliefs, and narratives that are more effective than ineffective, habitual thoughts and beliefs
- Understanding the role of trauma in chronic pain and how to seek trauma treatment
- Healthy relationships and belonging
  - Identifying and changing old patterns that you bring to relationships
  - Setting boundaries in general and around chronic pain issues
  - Nurturing the good in relationships
  - Partnering with significant others to address your pain
  - Knowing how to spot unhealthy relationship dynamics
- Savoring
- Self-compassion
  - Kind friend practice
  - Inner child exercise
  - Being your own best friend
- Benefiting others
  - Acts of kindness
  - Volunteering
  - Chronic pain advocacy
- Meaning in life
  - Reflecting on core values
  - Aligning values and actions
- Healthy diet
  - The standard American diet as a threat that ramps up the immune system
  - General dietary recommendations for lowering chronic pain and inflammation
  - The importance of personalized nutrition

- Sleep hygiene principles and cognitive-behavioral therapy for insomnia (CBT-I)
  - Being smart about your exposure to light
  - Addressing racing thoughts
  - CBT-i Coach (a smartphone app for insomnia) and finding an insomnia treatment specialist
- Physical activity
  - Physical inactivity as a threat to our bodies
  - Pacing yourself
    - This may involve grieving what you've lost (the ability to just get up and go without thinking) and moving forward in ways that work for you
    - Movement snacks
    - The benefits of working with a trained professional (a physical therapist)
- Integrative pain care
  - There's a lot more out there besides pills, surgeries, and injections. Approaches like spinal manipulation, massage, photobiomodulation, and neuromodulation are complementary approaches that can be discussed in collaboration with your care team.

EXERCISE

Using all you've learned you can create an *upward spiral* for yourself. Dr. Barbara Fredrickson, a leading happiness researcher at the University of North Carolina, coined the term "upward spiral" in her compelling research on the importance of positive emotions to setting healthy patterns in motion. Each thing we do has the potential to favorably impact multiple areas of our lives and open new possibilities for growth and change. As you reflect on everything you've learned, consider filling out your own unique vision of an "upward spiral" toward pain reduction, happiness, and purpose using the graphic that follows.

List those things that feel most important, urgent, or fundamental to your own unique healing process at the bottom of the spiral. For instance, maybe you really are finally ready to let go of self-defeating thoughts that you're a burden or not enough. You're ready to notice them when they arise and trust that they're not really true. Maybe you want to commit to supporting your brain's reward system by practicing savoring for 20 minutes every day along with working on a creative project three days per week.

Maybe you intuit that adopting a healthy diet with the guidance of a dietitian is something you're lacking and that you're ready to try. List what you see as most important below (or in a journal) and consider how these different skills could work together and build on one another to set you on an upward spiral path. Next, I'll help you set some daily, weekly, and monthly goals.

My Upward Spiral

Things I'm ready to let go of	Pain reduction, happiness, and purpose	Things I want to do

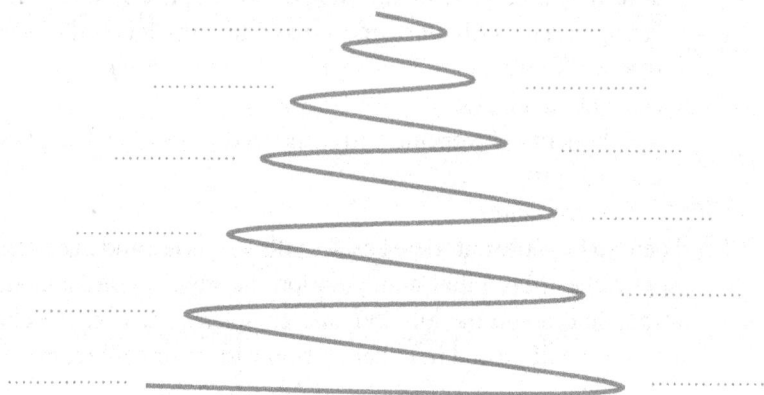

Consider sharing your spiral diagram, once you've completed it, with others you are close to who are involved in your chronic pain care.

Setting Goals

Once you have an idea of what you want to add to your life and let go of to create your holistic pain self-management plan, you can prepare to implement the plan by setting some goals. The best way to achieve your goals is to break down what you'll do by time period: day, week, month, and year. As you consider new goals, try to make them specific, measurable, and realistic.

A Typical Day

Start by brainstorming small changes that you can make daily. How would you like your typical day to be different than it is today? A few minutes of brain retraining and new behavior engagement per day adds up over weeks, months, and years.

Let's start with a **morning routine.** How do you want to start your day?

Examples: *Meditate for 5 minutes using a mindfulness app, spend 2 minutes savoring a cup of tea or coffee, and reflect on 2 things I'm grateful for. Walk the dog for 15 minutes. Remind myself of what's most meaningful to me and set an intention for the day. Identify what healthy meals and snacks I will eat during the day.*

My morning routine: ....

....

....

Think about a **midday routine.** How do you want to nourish yourself?

Examples: *Boost my reward system by taking a 30- to 45-minute walk during which I intentionally savor my surroundings. Lift weights for 30 minutes at the gym and eat a healthy, homemade lunch.*

My midday routine: ....

....

....

Consider **an evening routine** that will help your pain.

Examples: *Stop looking at my phone an hour before bed and dim the household lights. Build myself up by reminding myself of the things that I did do (versus what I struggled to or couldn't do) and remind myself of ways that I am safe (supports that are present in my life, positive experiences from the day). Mindfully cook dinner or read something uplifting that keeps me in touch with my values and purpose.*

My evening routine: ....

....

....

Consider adding in **wellness "snacks"** or breaks that you can take at regular intervals throughout the day. This might feel more fitting to you than formulating morning, midday, and evening routines (or you might do both).

Examples:

<u>Every 45 minutes:</u> *Get up and move (yoga, body weight exercises, physical therapy exercises) for 5–10 minutes. Take three long breaths and relax my shoulders with every exhale. Replace smartphone scrolling with _____ tension-reducing activity. Make sure I'm staying hydrated.*

<u>As needed:</u> *Notice and let go of pain-related worry. When tension builds, ground myself. Remind myself to notice and let go of old patterns that are no longer serving me, such as compulsively searching for health information online, blaming myself or others, believing thoughts that depict worst-case scenarios, or addictive behaviors.*

My well-being break: ....

....

....

....

....

....

....

<u>Reflect on what support you need from others or your environment to help you achieve the above.</u>

Examples: *Professionals I need to consult, adjustments I need to make with my housemates or family, sleep and wake times, work accommodations.*

I would inquire about: ....

....

....

....

....

....

....

Weekly Goals

Now consider what you want to do once a week to lower your pain.

Examples: *Grocery shop and meal prep healthy food. Do a longer exercise session outdoors. Connect with friends or neighbors in person or over the phone. Do a longer meditation session (45 minutes). Attend spiritual or religious services.*

What I want to do on a weekly basis:

1. ....
2. ....
3. ....
4. ....

Monthly Goals

Think about activities or skills that require more resources that you'd like to do once a month.

Examples: *Get a massage, go for a 4-hour hike, do a 45-minute lovingkindness meditation session. Volunteer at a local charity for 2–4 hours, engage with something beautiful (art, music) in a new way (museums, concerts), attend religious or spiritual services, see my chiropractor.*

What I want to do monthly:

1. ....
2. ....
3. ....
4. ....

One-Year Vision

Finally, envision where you will be in one year. Use the following prompts to affirm yourself and envision your future.

In one year, I hope to:

Have built the following regular habits: ....

....

Feel: ....

....

Think about: ....

....

Trust: ....

....

Embrace: ....

....

Accept: ....

....

Create: ....

....

    With that, you have much to look forward to. It's my true and heartfelt wish that this book has been of benefit to you. Trust in yourself. You're not alone in this struggle, and not a thing is "wrong" with you for having chronic pain. You are worthy of love, respect, and support. Remember that there's no such thing as a "pain patient," as pain is part of what makes us human, and it comes for everyone. You're battling one of the hardest fights that life offers up; you are so extraordinarily strong. My best and kindest wishes to you, friend. I'm proud of you. May you be well, strong, and at ease.

My Integrative Pain Care Plan:
For My Providers

Medications and supplements list (write down everything you're taking, including the name, dose, and how often you take it, including injections or infusions):

Questions I currently have about medications or supplements:

(continued)

165

My Integrative Pain Care Plan *(page 2 of 4)*

Pain management approaches (other than medications and supplements) that I'm currently using (include EVERYTHING, from conventional treatments to complementary approaches):

Treatment/activity: ....

Provider name and contact: ....

Frequency and duration: ....

Questions and notes: ....

Treatment/activity: ....

Provider name and contact: ....

Frequency and duration: ....

Questions and notes: ....

Treatment/activity: ....

Provider name and contact: ....

Frequency and duration: ....

Questions and notes: ....

Treatment/activity: ....

Provider name and contact: ....

Frequency and duration: ....

Questions and notes: ....

Treatment/activity: ....

Provider name and contact: ....

Frequency and duration: ....

Questions and notes: ....

Treatment/activity: ....

Provider name and contact: ....

Frequency and duration: ....

Questions and notes: ....

(continued)

Treatment/activity: ....

Provider name and contact: ....

Frequency and duration: ....

Questions and notes: ....

Treatments I Might Want to Try

Pain management approaches (other than medications and supplements) that I want to try or learn more about:

Treatment/activity: ....

Pros and cons: ....

Recommended providers: ....

Costs and insurance: ....

Can I get a letter of medical necessity? ....

Notes: ....

....

Pain management approaches (other than medications and supplements) that I want to try or learn more about:

Treatment/activity: ....

Pros and cons: ....

Recommended providers: ....

Costs and insurance: ....

Can I get a letter of medical necessity? ....

Notes: ....

....

Pain management approaches (other than medications and supplements) that I want to try or learn more about:

Treatment/activity: ....

Pros and cons: ....

Recommended providers: ....

Costs and insurance: ....

(continued)

My Integrative Pain Care Plan *(page 4 of 4)*

Can I get a letter of medical necessity? ....

Notes: ....

....

Pain management approaches (other than medications and supplements) that I want to try or learn more about:

Treatment/activity: ....

Pros and cons: ....

Recommended providers: ....

Costs and insurance: ....

Can I get a letter of medical necessity? ....

Notes: ....

....

Pain management approaches (other than medications and supplements) that I want to try or learn more about:

Treatment/activity: ....

Pros and cons: ....

Recommended providers: ....

Costs and insurance: ....

Can I get a letter of medical necessity? ....

Notes: ....

....

Pain management approaches (other than medications and supplements) that I want to try or learn more about:

Treatment/activity: ....

Pros and cons: ....

Recommended providers: ....

Costs and insurance: ....

Can I get a letter of medical necessity? ....

Notes: ....

....

Resources

**LEARN ABOUT PAIN AND STAY UP-TO-DATE
ON NEW DEVELOPMENTS**

United States Association for the Study of Pain (USASP)
www.usasp.org

International Association for the Study of Pain (IASP)
www.iasp-pain.org

U.S. Pain Foundation
https://uspainfoundation.org

American Psychological Association, Pain Psychology
www.apa.org/topics/pain

LEARN ABOUT PAIN NEUROSCIENCE

Curable
www.curablehealth.com

Lin Health
www.lin.health

Understanding Pain in Less than Five Minutes, a brief video
www.youtube.com/watch?v=5KrUL8tOaQs

The Pain Psychology Center
www.painpsychologycenter.com

Explain Pain
www.noigroup.com/product/explain-pain-second-edition

Why You Hurt
https://whyyouhurt.com/index.htm

SLEEP

CBT-i Coach
https://mobile.va.gov/app/cbt-i-coach

Society of Behavioral Sleep Medicine
www.behavioralsleep.org

NUTRITION

Find a registered dietitian in the United States at
www.eatright.org/find-a-nutrition-expert

INTEGRATIVE PAIN CARE

The International Association for the Study of Pain Global Year for
Integrative Pain Care (factsheets, articles, and more)
www.iasp-pain.org/advocacy/global-year/integrative-pain-care

The National Center for Complementary and Integrative Health
www.nccih.nih.gov

LEARN MORE ABOUT PSYCHEDELICS

The Multidisciplinary Association for Psychedelic Studies
https://maps.org/about-maps/mission

The Johns Hopkins Center for Psychedelic and Consciousness Research
www.hopkinsmedicine.org/psychiatry/research/psychedelics-research

LEARN MORE ABOUT MEDICAL CANNABIS

Cannabis (Marijuana) and Cannabinoids: What You Need to Know
www.nccih.nih.gov/health/cannabis-marijuana-and-cannabinoids-what-you-need-to-know

LEARN MORE ABOUT NEUROMODULATION

Neuromodulation Facts: Sources and Citations from the U.S. Pain Foundation
https://uspainfoundation.org/neuromod-sources

LEARN MORE ABOUT CHIROPRACTIC CARE

Chiropractic: In Depth
www.nccih.nih.gov/health/chiropractic-in-depth

Spinal Manipulation: What You Need to Know
www.nccih.nih.gov/health/spinal-manipulation-what-you-need-to-know

LEARN MORE ABOUT ACUPUNCTURE

American Academy of Medical Acupuncture
https://medicalacupuncture.org

Acupuncture: Effectiveness and Safety
www.nccih.nih.gov/health/acupuncture-what-you-need-to-know

LEARN MORE ABOUT PHOTOBIOMODULATION

IASP factsheet: Photobiomodulation and Thermal Therapies
www.iasp-pain.org/resources/fact-sheets/photobiomodulation-and-thermal-therapies

LEARN MORE ABOUT FUNCTIONAL MEDICINE

The Institute for Functional Medicine
www.ifm.org

**PARTICIPATE IN CLINICAL TRIALS FUNDED
BY THE NATIONAL INSTITUTES OF HEALTH**

Find Helping to End Addiction Long-Term (HEAL)-Funded Pain
Management Clinical Trials
https://heal.nih.gov/research/clinical-research/pain-management-clinical-trials

FIND A COUNSELOR SPECIALIZING IN CHRONIC PAIN

Search for "pain psychologist" on therapist directories: Inclusive
Therapists, Psychology Today, TherapyDen, Zencare, or ZocDoc

Pain Reprocessing Therapy provider directory
www.painreprocessingtherapy.com/clinician-directory

Google "pain psychologist" in your area

SUPPORT GROUPS

U.S. Pain Foundation's Pain Connection program
https://painconnection.org/support-groups

American Chronic Pain Association
www.acpanow.com/support-groups.html

GET FINANCIAL HELP WITH MEDICAL BILLS

www.usa.gov/help-with-medical-bills

NURTURE YOUR SOCIAL HEALTH

Deepen intimate relationships: The Gottman Institute:
A Research-Based Approach to Relationships
www.gottman.com

Set healthy boundaries: Nedra Tawwab's book: *Set Boundaries,
Find Peace*
www.nedratawwab.com

VOLUNTEER

Find ways to volunteer: *www.volunteermatch.org*

AARP's Create the Good website
https://createthegood.aarp.org

Advocate for people living with chronic pain
https://uspainfoundation.org/volunteer

Immediate help for intimate partner violence: National Domestic
Violence Hotline at 800-799-7233, or text START to 88788.

Learn the signs of unhealthy relationships: The One Love Foundation
www.joinonelove.org/signs-unhealthy-relationship

Bibliography

Afari, N., Ahumada, S. M., Wright, L. J., Mostoufi, S., Golnari, G., Reis, V., & Cuneo, J. G. (2014). Psychological trauma and functional somatic syndromes: A systematic review and meta-analysis. *Psychosomatic Medicine*, 76(1), 2–11.

Ambrose, K. R., & Golightly, Y. M. (2015). Physical exercise as non-pharmacological treatment of chronic pain: Why and when. *Best Practice & Research. Clinical Rheumatology*, 29(1), 120–130.

Anno, K., Shibata, M., Ninomiya, T., Iwaki, R., Kawata, H., Sawamoto, R., . . . Hosoi, M. (2015). Paternal and maternal bonding styles in childhood are associated with the prevalence of chronic pain in a general adult population: The Hisayama Study. *BMC Psychiatry*, 15(1), 1–8.

Ashar, Y. K., Gordon, A., Schubiner, H., Uipi, C., Knight, K., Anderson, Z., . . . Wager, T. D. (2022). Effect of pain reprocessing therapy vs. placebo and usual care for patients with chronic back pain: A randomized clinical trial. *JAMA Psychiatry*, 79(1), 13–23.

Bazzichi, L., Rossi, A., Massimetti, G., Giannaccini, G., Giuliano, T., De Feo, F., . . . Bombardieri, S. (2007). Cytokine patterns in fibromyalgia and their correlation with clinical manifestations. *Clinical and Experimental Rheumatology*, 25(2), 225–230.

Beecher, H. (1947). Pain in men wounded in battle. *The Journal of Nervous and Mental Disease*, 105(5), 544.

Beidelschies, M., Alejandro-Rodriguez, M., Guo, N., Postan, A., Jones, T., Bradley, E., . . . Rothberg, M. B. (2021). Patient outcomes and costs associated with functional medicine-based care in a shared versus individual setting for patients with chronic conditions: A retrospective cohort study. *BMJ Open, 11*(4), e048294.

Beidelschies, M., Alejandro-Rodriguez, M., Ji, X., Lapin, B., Hanaway, P., & Rothberg, M. B. (2019). Association of the functional medicine model of care with patient-reported health-related quality-of-life outcomes. *JAMA Network Open, 2*(10), e1914017.

Berry, M. P., Lutz, J., Schuman-Olivier, Z., Germer, C., Pollak, S., Edwards, R. R., . . . Napadow, V. (2020). Brief self-compassion training alters neural responses to evoked pain for chronic low back pain: A pilot study. *Pain Medicine, 21*(10), 2172–2185.

Boer, C. G., Radjabzadeh, D., Medina-Gomez, C., Garmaeva, S., Schiphof, D., Arp, P., . . . van Meurs, J. B. (2019). Intestinal microbiome composition and its relation to joint pain and inflammation. *Nature Communications, 10*(1), 4881.

Boring, B. L., Maffly-Kipp, J., Mathur, V. A., & Hicks, J. A. (2022). Meaning in life and pain: The differential effects of coherence, purpose, and mattering on pain severity, frequency, and the development of chronic pain. *Journal of Pain Research, 15,* 299–314.

Bradt, J., Norris, M., Shim, M., Gracely, E. J., & Gerrity, P. (2016). Vocal music therapy for chronic pain management in inner-city African Americans: A mixed methods feasibility study. *Journal of Music Therapy, 53*(2), 178–206.

Bubic, A., Von Cramon, D. Y., & Schubotz, R. I. (2010). Prediction, cognition and the brain. *Frontiers in Human Neuroscience, 4,* 1–25.

Burini, R. C., Anderson, E., Durstine, J. L., & Carson, J. A. (2020). Inflammation, physical activity, and chronic disease: An evolutionary perspective. *Sports Medicine and Health Science, 2*(1), 1–6.

Butler, D. S., & Moseley, G. L. (2013). *Explain pain: Revised and updated.* Noigroup Publications.

Carson, J. W., Keefe, F. J., Lynch, T. R., Carson, K. M., Goli, V., Fras, A. M., & Thorp, S. R. (2005). Loving-kindness meditation for chronic low back pain: Results from a pilot trial. *Journal of Holistic Nursing, 23*(3), 287–304.

Celidwen, Y., Redvers, N., Githaiga, C., Calambás, J., Añaños, K., Chindoy, M. E., . . . Sacbajá, A. (2023). Ethical principles of traditional Indigenous medicine to guide western psychedelic research and practice. *The Lancet Regional Health–Americas, 18,* 00410–100410.

Chandan, J. S., Keerthy, D., Gokhale, K. M., Bradbury-Jones, C., Raza, K., Bandyopadhyay, S., . . . Nirantharakumar, K. (2021). The association between exposure to domestic abuse in women and the development of syndromes indicating central nervous system sensitization: A retrospective cohort study using UK primary care records. *European Journal of Pain, 25*(6), 1283–1291.

Chang, A. M., Aeschbach, D., Duffy, J. F., & Czeisler, C. A. (2015). Evening use of light-emitting eReaders negatively affects sleep, circadian timing, and next-morning alertness. *Proceedings of the National Academy of Sciences of the USA, 112*(4), 1232–1237.

Chapin, H. L., Darnall, B. D., Seppala, E. M., Doty, J. R., Hah, J. M., & Mackey, S. C. (2014). Pilot study of a compassion meditation intervention in chronic pain. *Journal of Compassionate Health Care, 1*(1), 1–12.

Cheng, K., Martin, L. F., Slepian, M. J., Patwardhan, A. M., & Ibrahim, M. M. (2021). Mechanisms and pathways of pain photobiomodulation: A narrative review. *The Journal of Pain, 22*(7), 763–777.

Coakley, R., & Schechter, N. (2013). Chronic pain is like . . . The clinical use of analogy and metaphor in the treatment of chronic pain in children. *Pediatric Pain Letter, 15*(1), 1–8.

Coan, J. A., Schaefer, H. S., & Davidson, R. J. (2006). Lending a hand: Social regulation of the neural response to threat. *Psychological Science, 17,* 1032–1039.

Curry, O. S., Rowland, L. A., Van Lissa, C. J., Zlotowitz, S., McAlaney, J., & Whitehouse, H. (2018). Happy to help? A systematic review and meta-analysis of the effects of performing acts of kindness on the well-being of the actor. *Journal of Experimental Social Psychology, 76,* 320–329.

Dezutter, J., Casalin, S., Wachholtz, A., Luyckx, K., Hekking, J., & Vandewiele, W. (2013). Meaning in life: An important factor for the psychological well-being of chronically ill patients. *Rehabilitation Psychology, 58*(4), 334–341.

Dezutter, J., Luyckx, K., & Wachholtz, A. (2015). Meaning in life in chronic pain patients over time: Associations with pain experience and psychological well-being. *Journal of Behavioral Medicine, 38,* 384–396.

Dompe, C., Moncrieff, L., Matys, J., Grzech-Leśniak, K., Kocherova, I., Bryja, A., . . . Dyszkiewicz-Konwińska, M. (2020). Photobiomodulation—underlying mechanism and clinical applications. *Journal of Clinical Medicine, 9*(6), 1724.

Dragan, S., Şerban, M. C., Damian, G., Buleu, F., Valcovici, M., & Christodorescu, R. (2020). Dietary patterns and interventions to alleviate chronic pain. *Nutrients, 12*(9), 2510.

Dunn, E. W., Aknin, L. B., & Norton, M. I. (2008). Spending money on others promotes happiness. *Science, 319*(5870), 1687–1688.

Duraccio, K. M., Zaugg, K. K., Blackburn, R. C., & Jensen, C. D. (2021). Does iPhone night shift mitigate negative effects of smartphone use on sleep outcomes in emerging adults? *Sleep Health, 7*(4), 478–484.

Eckert, A. L., Pabst, K., & Endres, D. M. (2022). A Bayesian model for chronic pain. *Frontiers in Pain Research, 3,* 966034.

Edwards, R. R., Dworkin, R. H., Sullivan, M. D., Turk, D. C., & Wasan, A. D.

(2016). The role of psychosocial processes in the development and mainte-
nance of chronic pain. *The Journal of Pain, 17*(9), T70–T92.

Eisenberg, E., Morlion, B., Brill, S., & Häuser, W. (2022). Medicinal cannabis
for chronic pain: The Bermuda triangle of low-quality studies, countless
meta-analyses and conflicting recommendations. *European Journal of Pain,
26*(6), 1183–1185.

Elma, Ö., Brain, K., & Dong, H. J. (2022). The importance of nutrition as a
lifestyle factor in chronic pain management: A narrative review. *Journal of
Clinical Medicine, 11*(19), 5950.

Elvan, A., Cevik, S., Vatansever, K., & Erak, I. (2024). The association between
mobile phone usage duration, neck muscle endurance, and neck pain
among university students. *Scientific Reports, 14*(1), 20116.

Emerson, S. R., Kurti, S. P., Harms, C. A., Haub, M. D., Melgarejo, T., Logan,
C., & Rosenkranz, S. K. (2017). Magnitude and timing of the postprandial
inflammatory response to a high-fat meal in healthy adults: A systematic
review. *Advances in Nutrition, 8*(2), 213–225.

Ferrari, M., Hunt, C., Harrysunker, A., Abbott, M. J., Beath, A. P., & Einstein,
D. A. (2019). Self-compassion interventions and psychosocial outcomes: A
meta-analysis of RCTs. *Mindfulness, 10*, 1455–1473.

Field, R., Pourkazemi, F., Turton, J., & Rooney, K. (2021). Dietary interventions
are beneficial for patients with chronic pain: A systematic review with
meta-analysis. *Pain Medicine, 22*(3), 694–714.

Fifi, A. C., & Holton, K. F. (2020). Food in chronic pain: Friend or foe? *Nutrients, 12*(8), 2473.

Finlay, K. A., Peacock, S., & Elander, J. (2018). Developing successful social
support: An interpretative phenomenological analysis of mechanisms and
processes in a chronic pain support group. *Psychology & Health, 33*(7),
846–871.

Fischer, C. P., Berntsen, A., Perstrup, L. B., Eskildsen, P., & Pedersen, B. K.
(2007). Plasma levels of interleukin-6 and C-reactive protein are associated with physical inactivity independent of obesity. *Scandinavian Journal
of Medicine & Science in Sports, 17*(5), 580–587.

Fisher, J. P., Hassan, D. T., & O'Connor, N. (1995). Minerva. *British Medical
Journal, 310*, 70.

Fitzmaurice, B., Heneghan, N. R., Rayen, A., & Soundy, A. (2022). Whole-
body photobiomodulation therapy for chronic pain: A protocol for a feasibility trial. *BMJ Open, 12*(6), e060058.

Floyd, K., Mikkelson, A. C., Tafoya, M. A., Farinelli, L., La Valley, A. G., Judd,
J., . . . Wilson, J. (2007). Human Affection Exchange: XIII. Affectionate
communication accelerates neuroendocrine stress recovery. *Health Communication, 22*(2), 123–132.

Frankl, V. E. (1959). *Man's search for meaning*. Beacon Press.

Fredrickson, B. L., & Joiner, T. (2002). Positive emotions trigger upward spirals toward emotional well-being. *Psychological Science, 13*(2), 172–175.

Frey, P.-E., & Schiltenwolf, M. (2022). Chronic pain and exercise. *Deutsche Zeitschrift Für Sportmedizin, 73*(3), 98–105.

Garland, E. L. (2016). Restructuring reward processing with Mindfulness-Oriented Recovery Enhancement: Novel therapeutic mechanisms to remediate hedonic dysregulation in addiction, stress, and pain. *Annals of the New York Academy of Sciences, 1373*(1), 25–37.

Garland, E. L. (2020). Psychosocial intervention and the reward system in pain and opioid misuse: New opportunities and directions. *Pain, 161*(12), 2659.

Garland, E. L., Fix, S. T., Hudak, J. P., Bernat, E. M., Nakamura, Y., Hanley, A. W., . . . Froeliger, B. (2023). Mindfulness-Oriented Recovery Enhancement remediates anhedonia in chronic opioid use by enhancing neurophysiological responses during savoring of natural rewards. *Psychological Medicine, 53*(5), 2085–2094.

Garza-Villarreal, E. A., Wilson, A. D., Vase, L., Brattico, E., Barrios, F. A., Jensen, T. S., . . . Vuust, P. (2014). Music reduces pain and increases functional mobility in fibromyalgia. *Frontiers in Psychology, 5*, 90.

Gatchel, R. J., Reuben, D. B., Dagenais, S., Turk, D. C., Chou, R., Hershey, A. D., . . . Horn, S. D. (2018). Research agenda for the prevention of pain and its impact: Report of the work group on the prevention of acute and chronic pain of the Federal Pain Research Strategy. *The Journal of Pain, 19*(8), 837–851.

Geneen, L. J., Moore, R. A., Clarke, C., Martin, D., Colvin, L. A., Smith, B. H., & Geneen, L. J. (2017). Physical activity and exercise for chronic pain in adults: An overview of Cochrane Reviews. *Cochrane Database of Systematic Reviews, 2020*(2), CD011279.

Gleeson, M., Bishop, N. C., Stensel, D. J., Lindley, M. R., Mastana, S. S., & Nimmo, M. A. (2011). The anti-inflammatory effects of exercise: Mechanisms and implications for the prevention and treatment of disease. *Nature Reviews Immunology, 11*(9), 607–615.

Gorovoy, S. B., Campbell, R. L., Fox, R. S., & Grandner, M. A. (2023). App-supported sleep coaching: Implications for sleep duration and sleep quality. *Frontiers in Sleep, 2*, 1156844.

Griffiths, R. R., Johnson, M. W., Carducci, M. A., Umbricht, A., Richards, W. A., Richards, B. D., . . . Klinedinst, M. A. (2016). Psilocybin produces substantial and sustained decreases in depression and anxiety in patients with life-threatening cancer: A randomized double-blind trial. *Journal of Psychopharmacology, 30*(12), 1181–1197.

Gruszczyńska, E., & Knoll, N. (2015). Meaning-focused coping, pain, and affect:

A diary study of hospitalized women with rheumatoid arthritis. *Quality of Life Research, 24*(12), 2873–2883.

Hanh, T. N. (2017). *The art of living: Peace and freedom in the here and now.* HarperCollins.

Hanley, A. W., Nakamura, Y., & Garland, E. L. (2018). The Nondual Awareness Dimensional Assessment (NADA): New tools to assess nondual traits and states of consciousness occurring within and beyond the context of meditation. *Psychological Assessment, 30*(12), 1625–1639.

Hansen, M. M., Jones, R., & Tocchini, K. (2017). Shinrin-yoku (forest bathing) and nature therapy: A state-of-the-art review. *International Journal of Environmental Research and Public Health, 14*(8), 851.

Häuser, W., Finn, D. P., Kalso, E., Krcevski-Skvarc, N., Kress, H. G., Morlion, B., . . . Brill, S. (2018). European Pain Federation (EFIC) position paper on appropriate use of cannabis-based medicines and medical cannabis for chronic pain management. *European Journal of Pain, 22*, 1547–1564.

Hayes, S. C., Strosahl, K. D., & Wilson, K. G. (2016). *Acceptance and commitment therapy: The process and practice of mindful change* (2nd ed.). Guilford Press.

Henschke, N., Maher, C. G., Refshauge, K. M., Herbert, R. D., Cumming, R. G., Bleasel, J., . . . McAuley, J. H. (2009). Prevalence of and screening for serious spinal pathology in patients presenting to primary care settings with acute low back pain. *Arthritis & Rheumatism: Official Journal of the American College of Rheumatology, 60*(10), 3072–3080.

Hunt, C., Lerman, S. F., Smith, K., Keaser, M. L., Bingham, C., Zeidan, F., . . . Finan, P. H. (2022). Brief training in savoring meditation enhances non-dual awareness in rheumatoid arthritis patients. *The Journal of Pain, 23*(5), 55.

Hunt, C. A., Smith, M. T., Mun, C. J., Irwin, M. R., & Finan, P. H. (2021). Trait positive affect buffers the association between experimental sleep disruption and inflammation. *Psychoneuroendocrinology, 129*, 105240.

Hunter, K. (2023, June 16). *How to deal with racial trauma, according to Black experts.* Vox. *www.vox.com/even-better/23739289/racial-chronic-stress-trauma-help-mental-health*

Hysing, E. B., Smith, L., Thulin, M., Karlsten, R., Bothelius, K., & Gordh, T. (2019). Detection of systemic inflammation in severely impaired chronic pain patients and effects of a multimodal pain rehabilitation program. *Scandinavian Journal of Pain, 19*(2), 235–244.

The Institute for Molecular Bioscience at The University of Queensland (2019). Inflammation: The latest in research and discovery. *The Edge.* *https://imb.uq.edu.au/files/28591/The-Edge-Inflammation-IMB-UQ.pdf?utm_medium=website&utm_campaign=landingpagebottomBTN*

International Association for the Study of Pain. (2020). *The why, what and how of nutrition for people experiencing chronic pain*. [Video]. YouTube. *www.youtube.com/watch?v=gZusSZnxITc*

International Association for the Study of Pain. (2021, March 18). *IASP Position Statement on the Use of Cannabinoids to Treat Pain*. *www.iasp-pain.org/publications/iasp-news/iasp-position-statement-on-the-use-of-cannabinoids-to-treat-pain*

Irwin, M. R., & Olmstead, R. (2012). Mitigating cellular inflammation in older adults: A randomized controlled trial of tai chi. *The American Journal of Geriatric Psychiatry, 20*(9), 764–772.

Jensen, M. C., Brant-Zawadzki, M. N., Obuchowski, N., Modic, M. T., Malkasian, D., & Ross, J. S. (1994). Magnetic resonance imaging of the lumbar spine in people without back pain. *New England Journal of Medicine, 331*(2), 69–73.

Jiang-Xie, L.-F., Drieu, A., Bhasiin, K., Quintero, D., Smirnov, I., & Kipnis, J. (2024). Neuronal dynamics direct cerebrospinal fluid perfusion and brain clearance. *Nature, 627*(8002), 157–164.

Johnson, K. V.-A., & Dunbar, R. I. M. (2016). Pain tolerance predicts human social network size. *Scientific Reports, 6*(1), 25267.

Johnson, M. I. (2019). The landscape of chronic pain: Broader perspectives. *Medicina, 55*(5), 182.

Johnson, M. W., & Griffiths, R. R. (2017). Potential therapeutic effects of psilocybin. *Neurotherapeutics, 14*, 734–740.

Kandola, A., Ashdown-Franks, G., Hendrikse, J., Sabiston, C. M., & Stubbs, B. (2019). Physical activity and depression: Towards understanding the antidepressant mechanisms of physical activity. *Neuroscience & Biobehavioral Reviews, 107*, 525–539.

Kaptchuk, T. J., & Miller, F. G. (2018). Open label placebo: Can honestly prescribed placebos evoke meaningful therapeutic benefits? *BMJ, 363*, k3889.

Karos, K. (2022). Discrimination as one of the social plights facing people with pain. *Pain, 163*(2), e149–e150.

Kennedy, B. (2022). *Good Inside: A Guide to Becoming the Parent You Want to Be*. HarperCollins.

Khan, C. M., Iida, M., Stephens, M. A. P., Fekete, E. M., Druley, J. A., & Greene, K. A. (2009). Spousal support following knee surgery: Roles of self-efficacy and perceived emotional responsiveness. *Rehabilitation Psychology, 54*(1), 28.

Kolton, K. P. (2000). Analgesia following exercise: A review. *Sports Medicine, 29*(2), 85–98.

Lambert, G. W., Reid, C., Kaye, D. M., Jennings, G. L., & Esler, M. D. (2002). Effect of sunlight and season on serotonin turnover in the brain. *The Lancet, 360*(9348), 1840–1842.

Landmark, T., Romundstad, P., Borchgrevink, P. C., Kaasa, S., & Dale, O. (2011). Associations between recreational exercise and chronic pain in the general population: Evidence from the HUNT 3 study. *Pain, 152*(10), 2241–2247.

Li, D., & Sullivan, W. C. (2016). Impact of views to school landscapes on recovery from stress and mental fatigue. *Landscape and Urban Planning, 148,* 149–158.

Li, Q., Morimoto, K., Nakadai, A., Inagaki, H., Katsumata, M., Shimizu, T., . . . Kawada, T. (2007). Forest bathing enhances human natural killer activity and expression of anti-cancer proteins. *International Journal of Immunopathology and Pharmacology, 20*(2 Suppl. 2), 3–8.

Lipton, R. B., Dodick, D. W., Silberstein, S. D., Saper, J. R., Aurora, S. K., Pearlman, S. H., . . . Goadsby, P. J. (2010). Single-pulse transcranial magnetic stimulation for acute treatment of migraine with aura: A randomised, double-blind, parallel-group, sham-controlled trial. *Lancet Neurology, 9*(4), 373–380.

Lu, H. C., & Mackie, K. (2021). Review of the endocannabinoid system. *Biological Psychiatry: Cognitive Neuroscience and Neuroimaging, 6*(6), 607–615.

Lutz, J., Berry, M. P., Napadow, V., Germer, C., Pollak, S., Gardiner, P., . . . Schuman-Olivier, Z. (2020). Neural activations during self-related processing in patients with chronic pain and effects of a brief self-compassion training–a pilot study. *Psychiatry Research: Neuroimaging, 304,* 111155.

Maeda, Y., Kim, H., Kettner, N., Kim, J., Cina, S., Malatesta, C., . . . Napadow, V. (2017). Rewiring the primary somatosensory cortex in carpal tunnel syndrome with acupuncture. *Brain, 140*(4), 914–927.

Maher, C., Underwood, M., & Buchbinder, R. (2017). Non-specific low back pain. *The Lancet, 389* (10070), 736–747.

Manninen, S., Tuominen, L., Dunbar, R. I., Karjalainen, T., Hirvonen, J., Arponen, E., . . . Nummenmaa, L. (2017). Social laughter triggers endogenous opioid release in humans. *Journal of Neuroscience, 37*(25), 6125–6131.

Marion-Letellier, R., Amamou, A., Savoye, G., & Ghosh, S. (2019). Inflammatory bowel diseases and food additives: To add fuel on the flames. *Nutrients, 11*(5), 1111.

Martin, L. F., Patwardhan, A. M., Jain, S. V., Salloum, M. M., Freeman, J., Khanna, R., . . . Ibrahim, M. M. (2021). Evaluation of green light exposure on headache frequency and quality of life in migraine patients: A preliminary one-way cross-over clinical trial. *Cephalalgia, 41*(2), 135–147.

Martinez-Calderon, J., García-Muñoz, C., Rufo-Barbero, C., Matias-Soto, J., & Cano-García, F. J. (2024). Acceptance and commitment therapy for chronic pain: An overview of systematic reviews with meta-analysis of randomized clinical trials. *The Journal of Pain, 25*(3), 595–617.

Mayer, E. A., & Burns, T. (2016). *The mind-gut connection: How the hidden conversation within our bodies impacts our mood, our choices, and our overall health.* Harper Wave.

McBeth, J., Pye, S. R., O'Neill, T. W., Macfarlane, G. J., Tajar, A., Bartfai, G., . . . Wu, F. C. W. (2010). Musculoskeletal pain is associated with very low levels of vitamin D in men: Results from the European Male Ageing Study. *Annals of the Rheumatic Diseases, 69*(8), 1448–1452.

McWilliams, L. A., Cox, B. J., & Enns, M. W. (2000). Impact of adult attachment styles on pain and disability associated with arthritis in a nationally representative ample. *The Clinical Journal of Pain, 16*(4), 360–364.

Meredith, P., Ownsworth, T., & Strong, J. (2008). A review of the evidence linking adult attachment theory and chronic pain: Presenting a conceptual model. *Clinical Psychology Review, 28*(3), 407–429.

Mirgain, S. A. & Singles, J. (2016). *Self-management of chronic pain.* Whole Health Library, U.S. Department of Veterans Affairs. *www.va.gov/ WHOLEHEALTHLIBRARY/overviews/self-management-chronic-pain.asp*

Moseley, G. L., & Arntz, A. (2007). The context of a noxious stimulus affects the pain it evokes. *Pain, 133*(1–3), 64–71.

Moseley, G. L., & Butler, D. S. (2015). Fifteen years of explaining pain: The past, present, and future. *The Journal of Pain, 16*(9), 807–813.

Mostafalou, S., & Abdollahi, M. (2013). Pesticides and human chronic diseases: Evidences, mechanisms, and perspectives. *Toxicology and Applied Pharmacology, 268*(2), 157–177.

Müller, R., Segerer, W., Ronca, E., Gemperli, A., Stirnimann, D., Scheel-Sailer, A., & Jensen, M. P. (2022). Inducing positive emotions to reduce chronic pain: A randomized controlled trial of positive psychology exercises. *Disability and Rehabilitation, 44*(12), 2691–2704.

Myers, I. (2024, February 29). *EWG's dirty dozen guide to food chemicals: The top 12 to avoid.* EWG. *www.ewg.org/consumer-guides/ewgs-dirty-dozen-guide-food-chemicals-top-12-avoid*

Nahin, R. L., Rhee, A., & Stussman, B. (2024). Use of complementary health approaches overall and for pain management by US adults. *JAMA, 331*(7), 613–615.

Napadow, V. (2018). When a white horse is a horse: Embracing the (obvious?) overlap between acupuncture and neuromodulation. *The Journal of Alternative and Complementary Medicine, 24*(7), 621–623.

National Library of Medicine. (2024, May). *Facts about trans fats*. MedlinePlus. *https://medlineplus.gov/ency/patientinstructions/000786.htm*

Navratilova, E., & Porreca, F. (2014). Reward and motivation in pain and pain relief. *Nature Neuroscience, 17*(10), 1304–1312.

Neff, K. D. (2003). The development and validation of a scale to measure self-compassion. *Self and Identity, 2*(3), 223–250.

Nelson, S. K., Layous, K., Cole, S. W., & Lyubomirsky, S. (2016). Do unto others or treat yourself? The effects of prosocial and self-focused behavior on psychological flourishing. *Emotion, 16*(6), 850–861.

Nguyen, N. P., Kim, S. Y., Daheim, J., & Neduvelil, A. (2020). Social contribution and psychological well-being among midlife adults with chronic pain: A longitudinal approach. *Journal of Aging and Health, 32*(10), 1591–1601.

Nijs, J., Malfliet, A., Roose, E., Lahousse, A., Van Bogaert, W., Johansson, E., . . . Huysmans, E. (2024). Personalized multimodal lifestyle intervention as the best-evidenced treatment for chronic pain: State-of-the-art clinical perspective. *Journal of Clinical Medicine, 13*(3), 644.

Niruthisard, S., Ma, Q., & Napadow, V. (2023). *Acupuncture for pain relief.* IASP 2023 Global Year for Integrative Pain Care. *https://www.iasp-pain. org/resources/fact-sheets/acupuncture-for-pain-relief*

Nixon, A. E., Mazzola, J. J., Bauer, J., Krueger, J. R., & Spector, P. E. (2011). Can work make you sick? A meta-analysis of the relationships between job stressors and physical symptoms. *Work & Stress, 25*(1), 1–22.

Oaklander, M. (2016, April 28). "Why Friends Are Better Than Morphine." *TIME. https://time.com/4310991/friends-pain-morphine*

O'Connor, S. R., Tully, M. A., Ryan, B., Bleakley, C. M., Baxter, G. D., Bradley, J. M., & McDonough, S. M. (2015). Walking exercise for chronic musculoskeletal pain: Systematic review and meta-analysis. *Archives of Physical Medicine and Rehabilitation, 96*(4), 724–734.e3.

Paras, M. L., Murad, M. H., Chen, L. P., Goranson, E. N., Sattler, A. L., Colbenson, K. M., . . . Zirakzadeh, A. (2009). Sexual abuse and lifetime diagnosis of somatic disorders: A systematic review and meta-analysis. *JAMA, 302*(5), 550–561.

Park, J. W., & Chung, J. W. (2016). Inflammatory cytokines and sleep disturbance in patients with temporomandibular disorders. *Journal of Oral & Facial Pain and Headache, 30*(1), 27–33.

Peckover, S. (2002). Domestic abuse and women's health: The challenge for primary care. *Primary Health Care Research & Development, 3*(3), 151–158.

Pfeifer, A.-C., Ehrenthal, J. C., Neubauer, E., Gerigk, C., & Schiltenwolf, M. (2016). Impact of attachment behavior on chronic and somatoform pain. *Schmerz, 30*(5), 444–456.

Philpot, U. & Johnson, M. I. (2019). Diet therapy in the management of chronic pain: Better diet less pain? *Pain Management, 9*(4), 335–338.

Poulin, M. J., & Holman, E. A. (2013). Helping hands, healthy body? Oxytocin receptor gene and prosocial behavior interact to buffer the association between stress and physical health. *Hormones and Behavior, 63*(3), 510–517.

Purdie, F., & Morley, S. (2016). Compassion and chronic pain. *Pain, 157*(12), 2625–2627.

Romeo, A., Tesio, V., Castelnuovo, G., & Castelli, L. (2017). Attachment style and chronic pain: Toward an interpersonal model of pain. *Frontiers in Psychology, 8*, 284.

Rondanelli, M., Faliva, M. A., Miccono, A., Naso, M., Nichetti, M., Riva, A., . . . Perna, S. (2018). Food pyramid for subjects with chronic pain: Foods and dietary constituents as anti-inflammatory and antioxidant agents. *Nutrition Research Reviews, 31*(1), 131–151.

Salimpoor, V. N., Zatorre, R. J., Benovoy, M., Larcher, K., & Dagher, A. (2011). Anatomically distinct dopamine release during anticipation and experience of peak emotion to music. *Nature Neuroscience, 14*(2), 257–262.

Scott, W., Jackson, S. E., & Hackett, R. A. (2022). Perceived discrimination, health, and well-being among adults with and without pain: A prospective study. *Pain, 163*(2), 258–266.

Slade, G. D., Conrad, M. S., Diatchenko, L., Rashid, N. U., Zhong, S., Smith, S., . . . Nackley, A. G. (2011). Cytokine biomarkers and chronic pain: Association of genes, transcription, and circulating proteins with temporomandibular disorders and widespread palpation tenderness. *Pain, 152*(12), 2802–2812.

Slatcher, R. B., & Selcuk, E. (2017). A social psychological perspective on the links between close relationships and health. *Current Directions in Psychological Science, 26*(1), 16–21.

Stenberg, N., Gillison, F., & Rodham, K. (2022). How do peer support interventions for the self-management of chronic pain, support basic psychological needs? A systematic review and framework synthesis using self-determination theory. *Patient Education and Counseling, 105*(11), 3225–3234.

Stewart, L. K., Flynn, M. G., Campbell, W. W., Craig, B. A., Robinson, J. P., Timmerman, K. L., . . . Talbert, E. (2007). The influence of exercise training on inflammatory cytokines and C-reactive protein. *Medicine and Science in Sports and Exercise, 39*(10), 1714–1719.

Stults-Kolehmainen, M. A. (2023). Humans have a basic physical and psychological need to move the body: Physical activity as a primary drive. *Frontiers in Psychology, 14*, 1134049.

Tabor, A., Thacker, M. A., Moseley, G. L., & Körding, K. P. (2017). Pain: A statistical account. *PLOS Computational Biology, 13*(1), e1005142.

Tan, L., Cicuttini, F. M., Fairley, J., Romero, L., Estee, M., Hussain, S. M., & Urquhart, D. M. (2022). Does aerobic exercise effect pain sensitisation in individuals with musculoskeletal pain? A systematic review. *BMC Musculoskeletal Disorders, 23*(1), 1–21.

Tankha, H., Lumley, M. A., Gordon, A., Schubiner, H., Uipi, C., Harris, J., . . . Ashar, Y. K. (2023). "I don't have chronic back pain anymore": Patient experiences in pain reprocessing therapy for chronic back pain. *The Journal of Pain, 24*(9), 1582–1593.

Tatta, J., Pignataro, R. M., Bezner, J. R., George, S. Z., & Rothschild, C. E. (2023). PRISM—Pain Recovery and Integrative Systems Model: A process-based cognitive-behavioral approach for physical therapy. *Physical Therapy, 103*(10), pzad077.

Taylor, L. E. V., Stotts, N. A., Humphreys, J., Treadwell, M. J., & Miaskowski, C. (2013). A biopsychosocial-spiritual model of chronic pain in adults with sickle cell disease. *Pain Management Nursing, 14*(4), 287–301.

Tick, H. (2023). *Nutrition, the microbiome, and pain*. [Video]. YouTube. *www.youtube.com/watch?v=1zhnJfZwRsw*

Tick, H., Nielsen, A., Pelletier, K. R., Bonakdar, R., Simmons, S., Glick, R., . . . Zador, V. (2018). Evidence-based nonpharmacologic strategies for comprehensive pain care: The consortium pain task force white paper. *Explore, 14*(3), 177–211.

Tremblay, I., & Sullivan, M. J. L. (2010). Attachment and pain outcomes in adolescents: The mediating role of pain catastrophizing and anxiety. *The Journal of Pain, 11*(2), 160–171.

U.S. Department of Health and Human Services. (2019, May). *Pain management best practices inter-agency task force report: Updates, gaps, inconsistencies, and recommendations. www.hhs.gov/opioids/prevention/pain-management-options/index.html*

VA Office of Patient Centered Care and Cultural Transformation. (n.d.). *Values. www.va.gov/WHOLEHEALTHLIBRARY/docs/Values.pdf*

van den Berg, R., Jongbloed, E. M., de Schepper, E. I. T., Bierma-Zeinstra, S. M. A., Koes, B. W., & Luijsterburg, P. A. J. (2018). The association between pro-inflammatory biomarkers and nonspecific low back pain: A systematic review. *The Spine Journal, 18*(11), 2140–2151.

Vanti, C., Andreatta, S., Borghi, S., Guccione, A. A., Pillastrini, P., & Bertozzi, L. (2019). The effectiveness of walking versus exercise on pain and function in chronic low back pain: A systematic review and meta-analysis of randomized trials. *Disability and Rehabilitation, 41*(6), 622–632.

Vigar, V., Myers, S., Oliver, C., Arellano, J., Robinson, S., & Leifert, C. (2019). A systematic review of organic versus conventional food consumption: Is there a measurable benefit on human health? *Nutrients, 12*(1), 7.

Wang, Y., Ge, J., Zhang, H., Wang, H., & Xie, X. (2020). Altruistic behaviors relieve physical pain. *Proceedings of the National Academy of Sciences of the USA, 117*(2), 950–958.

Wegner, A., Elsenbruch, S., Maluck, J., Grigoleit, J. S., Engler, H., Jäger, M., . . . Benson, S. (2014). Inflammation-induced hyperalgesia: Effects of timing, dosage, and negative affect on somatic pain sensitivity in human experimental endotoxemia. *Brain, Behavior, and Immunity, 41*, 46–54.

White, A., Hayhoe, S., Hart, A., & Ernst, E. (2001). Adverse events following acupuncture: Prospective survey of 32,000 consultations with doctors and physiotherapists. *BMJ, 323*(7311), 485–486.

Yaden, D. B., Haidt, J., Hood, R. W., Vago, D. R., & Newberg, A. B. (2017). The varieties of self-transcendent experience. *Review of General Psychology, 21*(2), 143–160.

Yang, S., & Chang, M. C. (2020). Effect of repetitive transcranial magnetic stimulation on pain management: A systematic narrative review. *Frontiers in Neurology, 11*, 507027.

Zajacova, A., Grol-Prokopczyk, H., & Zimmer, Z. (2021). Pain trends among American adults, 2002–2018: Patterns, disparities, and correlates. *Demography, 58*(2), 711–738.

Zhang, M., Zhang, Y., Mu, Y., Wei, Z., & Kong, Y. (2021). Gender discrimination facilitates fMRI responses and connectivity to thermal pain. *NeuroImage, 244*, 118644.

Index

About the Author

Carly Hunt, PhD, is a Maryland-based health and performance psychologist and expert in chronic pain self-management. She has a private psychotherapy and consulting practice specializing in helping people optimize their health, well-being, and performance. She is also a Research Psychologist in the Johns Hopkins Department of Psychiatry and Behavioral Sciences. Dr. Hunt has lived with chronic pain and experienced the recovery process. She played college golf and continues to compete as an amateur locally and nationally.